THE ULTIMATE
LOW-FODMAP DIET
COOKBOOK FOR BEGINNERS

1100 Days of Simple & Delicious Recipes for Gut harmony,
Ibs Relief, and Digestive Wellbeing

MELISSA WESTWOOD

TABLE OF CONTENTS

Introduction

Welcome to your FODMAP journey, a road that can lead to a potentially life-changing understanding of your body, diet, and overall health. This journey is unique, and it's all about you – what you eat, how it affects your body, and how slight adjustments to your diet can significantly improve your quality of life.

Digestive discomfort is something millions of people face every day. If you're reading this book, you're likely one of them. Symptoms like bloating, stomach cramps, and irregular bowel movements can be distressing and even debilitating. Fortunately, you've taken the first step toward finding a solution – understanding the role of FODMAPs in your diet.

The FODMAP diet is not a traditional diet – it's not designed for weight loss, and it's not about counting calories. It's a dietary approach focused on managing digestive symptoms and promoting gut health. The journey won't always be easy. It may require patience, perseverance, and dedication, but the potential benefits are worthwhile.

The aim of this book is to guide you through your FODMAP journey, providing you with a deeper understanding of the diet, practical tips, and delicious low-FODMAP recipes. You'll find explanations of complex ideas in simple, accessible language, which will empower you to make informed decisions about your diet and health.

Understanding the Low-Fodmap Diet

FODMAP is an acronym that stands for Fermentable Oligosaccharides, Disaccharides, Monosaccharides, and Polyols. In simpler terms, FODMAPs are a group of carbohydrates that some people can't digest fully. They are found in a wide variety of foods, and when eaten, can lead to uncomfortable digestive symptoms in sensitive individuals.

Oligosaccharides are complex carbohydrates, and their name literally means "few sugars". Sounds harmless, right? Not so fast! These are the bad boys of the FODMAP family and include two subgroups: fructans and galacto-oligosaccharides (GOS). Their favorite hangout spots include wheat, rye, onions, garlic, and legumes. While they're quite popular in a variety of foods, these sneaky characters aren't easily absorbed by our gut, which can lead to some unwelcome digestive drama.

Next up, we have the Disaccharides, or "double sugars". The most infamous member of this group is lactose, found predominantly in milk and dairy products. If you've ever had an upset stomach after indulging in ice cream or a cheesy pizza, lactose might be your culprit. Our bodies need an enzyme called lactase to break down lactose, and for those of us who aren't blessed with enough of it, digesting these foods can feel like a mission impossible.

Polyols are found naturally in some fruits and vegetables and are commonly used as low-calorie sweeteners in "sugar-free" products. Their most well-known members are sorbitol and mannitol. These sugar alcohols might sound like a sweet deal, but unfortunately, they're not readily absorbed in our small intestine. The result? They can cause water to be drawn into the gut, leading to diarrhea for some people, or can become food for gut bacteria, resulting in gas and bloating for others. Double whammy!

Last but certainly not least, we have Monosaccharides, or "single sugars". The star player in this group is fructose, also known as fruit sugar. While fructose is found in a variety of fruits and sweeteners, not all fructose-containing foods are high in FODMAPs. It's only when the fructose outweighs glucose in a food that it becomes a FODMAP concern. An apple a day might not keep the doctor away if you're sensitive to fructose, as apples are higher in fructose than glucose.

The low-FODMAP diet is a two-phase approach developed by researchers at Monash University in Australia. It's primarily designed for those who suffer from Irritable Bowel Syndrome (IBS) and other digestive disorders.

The first phase, known as the elimination phase, involves removing all high-FODMAP foods from your diet for a few weeks. This gives your gut a chance to recover, and it allows you to observe whether your symptoms improve when these foods are not present.

The second phase, the reintroduction phase, involves gradually adding these foods back into your diet. This helps you to identify which FODMAPs you can tolerate, and in what quantities, with the ultimate goal of broadening your diet while managing your symptoms effectively.

Remember, the low-FODMAP diet is not about restricting your diet indefinitely but about identifying what triggers your symptoms so you can make more informed food choices. It's a journey towards a more personalized and comfortable way of eating.

It's essential to note that while this guide will provide you with comprehensive information, the FODMAP diet should ideally be undertaken under the guidance of a registered dietitian or healthcare professional experienced in this field. This will ensure that you maintain a balanced and nutritious diet while following the FODMAP diet plan.

Benefit of a Low Fodmap Diet

So, we've spent a fair amount of time chatting about your gut and how the low-FODMAP diet can be its new best buddy. We've talked about gas, bloating, and all things digestive, but are you ready for a plot twist? Hold onto your hat, because the low-FODMAP diet's benefits aren't just confined to the mysterious world of your digestive system. It's time to look beyond the belly and see what other tricks this diet has up its sleeve.

Enhanced Mental Well-being: Ever had a "gut-wrenching" experience or felt "butterflies in your stomach"? That's because your brain and gut are like two peas in a pod, constantly chatting with each other. When your gut is at peace, it can positively influence your mental health. Many individuals on a low-FODMAP diet report feeling less stressed and more cheerful. It's like the old saying goes: happy gut, happy life. Or something like that.

Better Sleep: When you embark on a low-FODMAP journey, one of the first things you might notice (apart from a quieter gut, of course) is the improvement in your sleep quality. With the symphony of rumbles and grumbles from your abdomen toned down, your trips to the bathroom reduce, leaving you with uninterrupted stretches of sleep. It's the difference between a fitful nap and a rejuvenating night's rest.

Research suggests that sleep disorders and gut health are tightly entwined. Poor gut health can lead to disrupted sleep, and conversely, insufficient sleep can wreak havoc on your gut. It's a vicious cycle, but one that a low-FODMAP diet might help you break.

Increased Energy: Many people on a low-FODMAP diet report feeling more energetic and less sluggish. If your body isn't constantly battling digestive distress, it's free to channel its energy elsewhere.

Feeling more energetic isn't just about being more productive, though. It's about enjoying life more fully. It's about having the energy to engage in spontaneous dance-offs with your neighbor or playing tag with your kids without getting winded. It's about being able to enjoy a sunset stroll or invest time in your hobbies without constantly checking your energy levels.

Weight Maintenance: While the low-FODMAP diet isn't a weight loss diet, eating balanced meals and paying attention to portion sizes can help with weight management. Plus, the increased energy levels might motivate you to stay active, indirectly contributing to maintaining a healthy weight.

Improved Nutrient Absorption: Certain gut issues can hinder the absorption of nutrients from food. By calming down your gut's temper tantrums, a low-FODMAP diet might aid in better nutrient absorption, ensuring your body gets the nourishment it needs.

When your body absorbs nutrients better, it's like upgrading from a dial-up connection to high-speed internet—everything just works better. You're not just consuming food; you're extracting all the wonderful nourishment it has to offer. Your cells get the fuel they need, your immune system gets the support it needs, and you get the health boost you need.

BREAKFAST RECIPES

FODMAP-Friendly Smoothie Bowl

Preparation time: 10 minutes

Cooking time: 0 minutes

Servings: 2

Ingredients:

- 2 cups (480 mL/60 grams) fresh spinach
- 1 cup (240 mL/245 grams) lactose-free yogurt
- 1 cup (240 mL/144 grams) fresh strawberries
- - 1 ripe banana (approx. 118 grams)
- - 2 tablespoons (30 mL/24 grams) chia seeds for topping

Directions:

1. Rinse the fresh spinach and strawberries under cold water.
2. Cut the strawberries into halves, and slice the banana.
3. Add the spinach, lactose-free yogurt, halved strawberries, and banana slices to a blender.
4. Blend until the mixture is smooth. If the smoothie is too thick, you can add a bit of water or lactose-free milk to reach your preferred consistency.
5. Pour the smoothie into two bowls.
6. Top each bowl with 1 tablespoon of chia seeds.
7. Serve immediately for the best taste and consistency.

Nutrition: Calories: 220; Fat: 6g; Carbs: 35g; Protein: 10g

Notes and Variations: - Feel free to add more toppings like a small serving of low-FODMAP fruits such as blueberries, raspberries, or orange slices. If you want to add a protein boost, sprinkle some hemp seeds on top. Remember to monitor your portion sizes.

Banana Pancakes

Preparation time: 10 minutes

Cooking time: 15 minutes

Servings: 2

Ingredients:

- 2 ripe bananas (about 240 grams)
- - 1 cup (240 mL/120 grams) gluten-free flour
- - 1/2 cup (120 mL/120 grams) almond milk
- - 1 teaspoon (5 mL/5 grams) baking powder
- - 1/4 teaspoon (1.25 mL/1.5 grams) salt
- - 1 tablespoon (15 mL/14 grams) vegetable oil (for cooking

Directions:

1. In a medium-sized bowl, mash the ripe bananas with a fork until it becomes a puree.
2. Add the gluten-free flour, almond milk, baking powder, and salt to the mashed bananas. Stir until well combined.
3. Heat a non-stick frying pan over medium heat and add a small amount of vegetable oil.
4. Pour about 1/4 cup (60 mL) of the pancake batter into the pan for each pancake.
5. Cook the pancakes for about 2-3 minutes on each side or until they are golden brown and cooked through. Repeat this process with the remaining batter.
6. Serve the pancakes warm with your choice of low FODMAP toppings, such as a drizzle of maple syrup or a sprinkle of cinnamon.

Nutrition: Calories: 400; Fat: 8g; Carbs: 80g; Protein: 8g

Notes and Variations: Remember to read labels when choosing a gluten-free flour, as some may contain high FODMAP ingredients. If the batter is too thick, add a bit more almond milk to reach your preferred consistency. Feel free to add some low FODMAP fruits on top for added flavor and nutrition. Just be mindful of the serving sizes to keep the meal low in FODMAPs.

Veggie Omelet

Preparation time: 10 minutes

Cooking time: 10 minutes

Servings: 1-2

Ingredients:

- 2 large eggs (about 100 grams)
- - 1/2 red bell pepper (about 75 grams), chopped
- - 1 cup fresh spinach (about 30 grams), chopped
- - 1/4 cup (60 mL/28 grams) cheddar cheese, grated
- - 1 tablespoon (15 mL/14 grams) olive oil
- - Salt and pepper to taste

Directions:

1. Crack the eggs into a bowl, season with a little salt and pepper, and beat them until the yolks and whites are fully combined.
2. Heat the olive oil in a non-stick frying pan over medium heat.
3. Add the chopped bell pepper to the pan and sauté for a couple of minutes until it starts to soften. Add the chopped spinach and continue to sauté until it wilts.
4. Pour the beaten eggs over the vegetables in the pan, tilting the pan slightly to spread them evenly.
5. Sprinkle the grated cheddar cheese on top of the eggs.
6. Cover the pan with a lid and let the omelet cook for a couple of minutes until the eggs are set and the cheese is melted.
7. Carefully fold the omelet in half using a spatula, then slide it onto a plate.

Nutrition: Calories: 320; Fat: 25g; Carbs: 5g; Protein: 18g

Notes and Variations: You can vary the vegetables according to what you have on hand, just remember to choose low FODMAP options. If you like your omelet more well-done, you can flip it over after adding the cheese and cook for an additional minute. If you're sensitive to lactose, ensure you're using a lactose-free cheese or skip the cheese altogether.

Quinoa Porridge

Preparation time: 5 minutes

Cooking time: 20 minutes

Servings: 1-2

Ingredients:

- 1/2 cup (120 mL/85 grams) quinoa
- - 2 cups (480 mL/480 grams) almond milk
- - 1/2 teaspoon (2.5 mL/1.3 grams) ground cinnamon
- - 1 tablespoon (15 mL/21 grams) maple syrup (optional)

Directions:

1. Rinse the quinoa under cold water until the water runs clear.
2. In a medium-sized pot, combine the rinsed quinoa and almond milk.
3. Bring the mixture to a boil over medium-high heat. Once boiling, reduce the heat to low and let it simmer.
4. Cook the quinoa, stirring occasionally, for about 15-20 minutes, or until the quinoa is tender and has absorbed most of the almond milk.
5. Stir in the ground cinnamon and sweeten with maple syrup if desired.
6. Serve warm and enjoy!

Nutrition: Calories: 360; Fat: 9g; Carbs: 60g; Protein: 12g

Notes and Variations: Quinoa porridge can be a delightful substitute for traditional oatmeal for those on a low FODMAP diet. Feel free to add toppings like a small serving of low-FODMAP fruits or a sprinkle of chia seeds for an extra nutritional punch.

Gluten-Free Toast with Almond Butter

Preparation time: 5 minutes

Cooking time: 2 minutes

Servings: 1

Ingredients:

- 1 slice of gluten-free bread (about 30 grams)
- - 1 tablespoon (15 mL/16 grams) almond butter

Directions:

1. Toast the slice of gluten-free bread until it reaches your desired level of crispiness.
2. Spread the almond butter evenly across the toasted bread.
3. Enjoy immediately while the toast is still warm.

Nutrition: Calories: 200; Fat: 11g; Carbs: 22g; Protein: 5g

Notes and Variations: You can sprinkle a small amount of chia seeds or flax seeds on top for extra fiber and nutrition. You could add a few slices of a low FODMAP fruit like a banana on top if you want to make this into a more substantial breakfast.

Gluten-Free Banana Muffins

Preparation time: 10 minutes

Cooking time: 25 minutes

Servings: 12 muffins

Ingredients:

- - 1 cup (200 grams) ripe bananas, mashed (about 2 medium bananas)
- - 2 large eggs
- - 1/2 cup (100 grams) granulated sugar
- - 1/3 cup (80 mL) vegetable oil
- - 1 teaspoon (5 mL) pure vanilla extract
- - 2 cups (280 grams) gluten-free all-purpose flour

- - 1 teaspoon (5 grams) baking powder
- - 1/2 teaspoon (2.5 grams) baking soda
- - 1/4 teaspoon (1.5 grams) salt
- - 1/2 teaspoon (2.5 grams) ground cinnamon

Directions:

1. Preheat your oven to 350°F (175°C). Line a muffin tin with paper liners or lightly grease it.
2. In a large bowl, whisk together the mashed bananas, eggs, sugar, oil, and vanilla extract until well combined.
3. In a separate bowl, combine the gluten-free flour, baking powder, baking soda, salt, and cinnamon.
4. Gradually add the dry ingredients to the wet ingredients, stirring until just combined.
5. Scoop the batter into the prepared muffin tin, filling each cup about 2/3 full.
6. Bake for 20-25 minutes, or until a toothpick inserted into the center of a muffin comes out clean.
7. Let the muffins cool in the tin for 5 minutes, then transfer them to a wire rack to cool completely.

Nutrition: Calories: 160 (per muffin); Fat: 6g; Carbs: 25g; Protein: 3g

Notes and Variations: You can add a handful of low FODMAP nuts or seeds to the batter for added texture and nutrition. Pecans, walnuts, or chia seeds would all be great options. If you'd like, you can also add a sprinkle of cinnamon and sugar on top of each muffin before baking for a sweet, crunchy topping. These muffins can be stored in an airtight container at room temperature for up to 3 days, or in the refrigerator for up to a week. They can also be frozen for up to 3 months.

Rice Cakes with Peanut Butter

Preparation time: 5 minutes

Cooking time: 0 minutes

Servings: 1-2

Ingredients:

- 2 rice cakes (about 18 grams each)

- - 2 tablespoons (30 mL/32 grams) peanut butter

Directions:

1. Spread one tablespoon of peanut butter evenly over each rice cake.
2. Enjoy immediately for a crisp and satisfying snack.

Nutrition: Calories: 210; Fat: 14g; Carbs: 16g; Protein: 7g

Notes and Variations: For extra flavor and texture, you could top the peanut butter with a sprinkle of chia seeds or a few slices of a low FODMAP fruit like a strawberry or a small banana. Remember to use natural peanut butter with no added sugars or high FODMAP ingredients.

Fruit Salad

Preparation time: 10 minutes

Cooking time: 0 minutes

Servings: 1-2

Ingredients:

- 1/2 cup (120 mL/72 grams) strawberries, hulled and halved
- - 1/2 cup (120 mL/80 grams) seedless grapes, halved

- - 1/2 cup (120 mL/130 grams) oranges, peeled and segmented

Directions:

1. In a bowl, combine the strawberries, grapes, and orange segments.
2. Gently toss the fruit until it's well combined.
3. Serve immediately or refrigerate until ready to eat.

Nutrition: Calories: 120; Fat: 0g; Carbs: 30g; Protein: 2g

Notes and Variations: This fruit salad is refreshing on its own, but you could also serve it with a dollop of lactose-free yogurt for a more substantial breakfast or snack. Feel free to vary the fruits based on your tolerance and the low FODMAP serving sizes. For example, blueberries, cantaloupe, or pineapple could also be included.

A sprinkle of chia seeds or a drizzle of maple syrup can add a different flavor dimension to your fruit salad. Keep in mind that while these fruits are low FODMAP in the given amounts, combining multiple servings of low FODMAP foods can still lead to a high overall FODMAP load. Adjust serving sizes based on your individual tolerance.

Scrambled Eggs with Chives

Preparation time: 5 minutes

Cooking time: 5 minutes

Servings: 1-2

Ingredients:

- 2 large eggs (about 100 grams)
- - 1 tablespoon (15 mL/14 grams) lactose-free milk or almond milk
- - Salt and pepper to taste
- - 1 tablespoon (15 mL/14 grams) butter
- - 1 tablespoon (3 grams) fresh chives, finely chopped

Directions:

1. In a bowl, whisk together the eggs, milk, salt, and pepper until well combined.
2. Melt the butter in a non-stick skillet over medium heat.
3. Pour the egg mixture into the skillet. As the eggs start to set, gently pull them across the pan with a spatula, forming soft curds.
4. Continue cooking - pulling, lifting and folding eggs - until thickened and no visible liquid egg remains. Be careful not to overcook.
5. Remove from heat and sprinkle with the chopped chives.
6. Serve immediately while still hot.

Nutrition: Calories: 210; Fat: 17g; Carbs: 1g; Protein: 12g

Notes and Variations: For a different flavor profile, you could substitute chives with other low FODMAP herbs like parsley or dill. If you can tolerate cheese, a sprinkle of grated cheddar or a dollop of lactose-free cream cheese could add a rich, creamy dimension to your scrambled eggs.

Always pay attention to how your body reacts to new foods introduced into your diet. It's important to listen to your body and adjust portion.

Remember, while eggs are a good source of protein and are low in FODMAPs, some people might still have sensitivities to them. If you suspect this might be the case for you, consult with a healthcare professional.

Quinoa Porridge
with Blueberries and Cinnamon

Preparation time: 5 minutes

Cooking time: 20 minutes

Servings: 1-2

Ingredients:

- 1/2 cup (120 mL/85 grams) uncooked quinoa
- - 1 cup (240 mL) almond milk
- - 1/2 teaspoon (2.5 mL/1.3 grams) cinnamon
- - 1/2 cup (120 mL/74 grams) blueberries

Directions:

1. Rinse the quinoa under cold water until the water runs clear. This removes any bitter tasting residue on the outside of the seeds.
2. In a saucepan, combine the rinsed quinoa and almond milk. Bring the mixture to a boil over medium-high heat.
3. Once boiling, reduce the heat to low, cover, and let simmer for 15-20 minutes, or until the quinoa has absorbed most of the liquid and is tender.
4. Stir in the cinnamon and blueberries. Cook for another 2-3 minutes, until the blueberries are warmed through.
5. Serve the quinoa porridge hot, with additional almond milk if desired.

Nutrition: Calories: 300; Fat: 5g; Carbs: 55g; Protein: 12g

Notes and Variations: For added sweetness, you could drizzle your quinoa porridge with a little bit of maple syrup or sprinkle with a small amount of brown sugar. However, remember to adjust your FODMAP count accordingly.

Banana Pancakes with Maple Syrup

Preparation time: 10 minutes

Cooking time: 10 minutes

Servings: 1-2

Ingredients:

- 1 medium ripe banana (about 120 grams)
- - 2 large eggs (about 100 grams)
- - 1/2 cup (120 mL/60 grams) gluten-free flour
- - 1/2 teaspoon (2.5 mL/2 grams) baking powder
- - 1/4 cup (60 mL) almond milk
- - Butter or oil for frying
- - 2 tablespoons (30 mL/40 grams) maple syrup

Directions:

1. .In a bowl, mash the ripe banana until smooth.
2. Add the eggs, gluten-free flour, baking powder, and almond milk to the mashed banana. Stir until all the ingredients are well combined.
3. Heat a non-stick skillet over medium heat. Add a small amount of butter or oil to the skillet.
4. Pour 1/4 cup of the pancake batter into the skillet. Cook for about 2-3 minutes, until the edges are set and bubbles form on the surface. Flip the pancake and cook for another 2-3 minutes on the other side.
5. Repeat with the remaining batter.
6. Serve the pancakes hot, drizzled with the maple syrup.

Nutrition: Calories: 410; Fat: 10g; Carbs: 70g; Protein: 14g

Notes and Variations: You could add a sprinkle of cinnamon to the pancake batter for an extra flavor twist. If you're looking for more texture in your pancakes, you could add a handful of low FODMAP nuts or seeds, such as walnuts or chia seeds. Be sure to adjust your FODMAP count accordingly.

Remember that ripe bananas are higher in FODMAPs than unripe ones. If you are in the elimination phase of the diet or know that you are sensitive to ripe bananas, you may want to substitute it with a FODMAP-safe serving of another fruit puree, like canned pumpkin.

Scrambled Eggs with Spinach and Feta

Preparation time: 5 minutes

Cooking time: 10 minutes

Servings: 1-2

Ingredients:

- 2 large eggs (about 100 grams)
- 1 tablespoon (15 mL/14 grams) lactose-free milk or almond milk
- Salt and pepper to taste
- 1 tablespoon (15 mL/14 grams) olive oil
- 1 cup (30 grams) fresh spinach
- - 1/4 cup (40 grams) Feta cheese, crumbled

Directions:

1. In a bowl, whisk together the eggs, milk, salt, and pepper until well combined.
2. Heat the olive oil in a non-stick skillet over medium heat.
3. Add the spinach to the skillet and sauté until wilted, about 1-2 minutes.

4. Pour the egg mixture over the spinach. As the eggs start to set, gently pull them across the pan with a spatula, forming soft curds.
5. When the eggs are almost set but still slightly runny, sprinkle the crumbled Feta cheese over the top. Allow the residual heat to melt the Feta slightly.
6. Serve immediately while still hot.

Nutrition: Calories: 285; Fat: 22g; Carbs: 3g; Protein: 17g

Notes and Variations: Feta cheese is low in lactose and is usually well-tolerated on a low FODMAP diet, but if you're sensitive to dairy or in the elimination phase of the diet, you could substitute it with a lactose-free cheese. Feel free to add other low FODMAP veggies to your scrambled eggs, like bell peppers or chives.

Rice Cakes with Peanut Butter and Banana Slices

Preparation time: 5 minutes	Cooking time: 0 minutes	Servings: 1-2

Ingredients:

- 2 plain rice cakes (about 14 grams each)
- - 2 tablespoons (30 mL/32 grams) natural peanut butter
- - 1/2 medium unripe banana (about 60 grams), sliced

Directions:

1. Spread 1 tablespoon of peanut butter over each rice cake.
2. Top each rice cake with banana slices.
3. Serve immediately and enjoy this quick, satisfying snack!

Nutrition: Calories: 240; Fat: 10g; Carbs: 30g; Protein: 8g

Notes and Variations: Natural peanut butter is usually a safe choice on the low FODMAP diet because it contains just peanuts and salt. Avoid peanut butter that contains added sugars or high FODMAP ingredients like honey or high fructose corn syrup. If you want to add a bit more flavor, you could sprinkle a dash of cinnamon on top of the banana slices.

Buckwheat Pancakes with Strawberries

Preparation time: 10 minutes	Cooking time: 15 minutes	Servings: 1-2

Ingredients:

- 1/2 cup (120 mL/65 grams) buckwheat flour
- - 1 teaspoon (5 mL/5 grams) baking powder
- - Pinch of salt
- - 1/2 cup (120 mL) lactose-free milk or almond milk
- - 1 large egg (about 50 grams)
- - 1 tablespoon (15 mL/14 grams) vegetable oil, plus extra for frying
- - 1/2 cup (75 grams) fresh strawberries, sliced 1

Directions:

1. In a bowl, combine the buckwheat flour, baking powder, and salt.
2. In another bowl, whisk together the milk, egg, and 1 tablespoon of oil.
3. Pour the wet ingredients into the dry ingredients and stir until just combined.
4. Heat a non-stick skillet over medium heat and add a small amount of oil.
5. Pour 1/4 cup of the pancake batter into the skillet. Cook for about 2-3 minutes, until the edges are set and bubbles form on the surface. Flip the pancake and cook for another 2-3 minutes on the other side.
6. Repeat with the remaining batter.
7. Serve the pancakes hot, topped with the sliced strawberries.

Nutrition: Calories: 395; Fat: 18g; Carbs: 50g; Protein: 14g

Notes and Variations: If you like your pancakes sweet, you could drizzle them with a small amount of pure maple syrup. Just remember to account for this in your FODMAP count.

If you're looking for a variation, try topping your pancakes with other low FODMAP fruits, like a small amount of blueberries or raspberries.

Smoked Salmon and Dill Omelette

Preparation time: 5 minutes

Cooking time: 10 minutes

Servings: 1-2

Ingredients:

- 2 large eggs (about 100 grams)
- - 2 tablespoons (30 mL/28 grams) lactose-free milk or almond milk
- - Salt and pepper to taste
- - 1 tablespoon (15 mL/14 grams) olive oil
- - 2 ounces (56 grams) smoked salmon, chopped
- - 1 tablespoon (1.6 grams) fresh dill, chopped

Directions:

1. In a bowl, whisk together the eggs, milk, salt, and pepper until well combined.

2. Heat the olive oil in a non-stick skillet over medium heat.
3. Pour the egg mixture into the skillet and allow it to cook undisturbed until it begins to set around the edges.
4. Sprinkle the smoked salmon and dill evenly over one half of the omelette.
5. Using a spatula, gently fold the omelette in half over the salmon and dill.
6. Continue to cook for another 2-3 minutes, or until the omelette is fully set and the salmon is heated through.
7. Slide the omelette onto a plate and serve immediately.

Nutrition: Calories: 325; Fat: 24g; Carbs: 2g; Protein: 24g

Notes and Variations: For added flavor, you could sprinkle a small amount of feta cheese over the salmon before folding the omelette. Just remember to account for this in your FODMAP count. If you're not a fan of dill, you could substitute it with chives or another low FODMAP herb of your choice.

Baked Frittata
with Bell Pepper and Cheddar

Preparation time: 10 minutes

Cooking time: 25 minutes

Servings: 1-2

Ingredients:

- 4 large eggs (about 200 grams)
- - 2 tablespoons (30 mL/28 grams) lactose-free milk or almond milk
- - Salt and pepper to taste
- - 1 tablespoon (15 mL/14 grams) olive oil
- - 1/2 medium green bell pepper (about 75 grams), diced
- - 1/2 medium red bell pepper (about 75 grams), diced
- - 1/4 cup (28 grams) cheddar cheese, shredded

Directions:

1. Preheat the oven to 375°F (190°C).
2. In a bowl, whisk together the eggs, milk, salt, and pepper until well combined.
3. Heat the olive oil in an oven-safe skillet over medium heat. Add the diced bell peppers and cook for about 5 minutes, until they start to soften.
4. Pour the egg mixture over the peppers in the skillet and stir gently to distribute the peppers evenly.
5. Sprinkle the shredded cheddar cheese over the top of the egg mixture.
6. Transfer the skillet to the preheated oven and bake for about 15-20 minutes, until the frittata is set and the cheese is golden.
7. Remove from the oven and let it cool for a few minutes before slicing and serving.

Nutrition: Calories: 415; Fat: 30g; Carbs: 9g; Protein: 28g

Notes and Variations: You can vary the vegetables used in this frittata based on what you have on hand and what you tolerate well. Other low FODMAP options could include spinach, tomatoes, or zucchini.

Gluten-Free Toast with Avocado and a Poached Egg

Preparation time: 10 minutes   Cooking time: 5 minutes   Servings: 1

Ingredients:

- 1 slice of gluten-free bread
- - 1/4 medium avocado (about 30 grams)
- - 1 large egg (about 50 grams)
- - Salt and pepper to taste
- - A pinch of paprika (optional)

Directions:

1. Start by toasting the gluten-free bread to your preferred level of crispness.
2. While the bread is toasting, bring a small pot of water to a boil. Once boiling, reduce the heat until the water is simmering.
3. Crack the egg into a small cup, then gently slide it into the simmering water. Allow it to cook for about 4 minutes for a runny yolk, or longer if you prefer a firmer yolk.
4. As the egg cooks, scoop out the avocado and mash it onto the toasted bread. Season it with a little salt and pepper.
5. When the egg is done, use a slotted spoon to carefully lift it out of the water. Let any excess water drip off, then place the egg on top of the avocado toast.
6. Season with a little more salt and pepper, and a sprinkle of paprika if desired. Serve immediately.

Nutrition: Calories: 250; Fat: 16g; Carbs: 20g; Protein: 10g

Notes and Variations: While avocados are not strictly low FODMAP, a small serving size of 30 grams is generally well tolerated by most people. You can add other low FODMAP toppings to this toast if you like. Some options could include a sprinkle of chia seeds, a drizzle of olive oil, or a few slices of tomato.

Blueberry and Almond Smoothie

Preparation time: 5 minutes   Cooking time: 0 minutes   Servings: 1

Ingredients:

- - 1/2 cup (70 grams) fresh or frozen blueberries
- - 1 cup (240 mL) unsweetened almond milk
- - 1 tablespoon (15 grams) almond butter
- - 1/2 medium banana (about 60 grams)
- - A handful of ice cubes

Directions:

1. Place all the ingredients in a blender.
2. Blend on high speed until smooth and creamy.
3. Pour the smoothie into a glass and serve immediately.

Nutrition: Calories: 230; Fat: 12g; Carbs: 30g; Protein: 5g

Notes and Variations: If you prefer a thicker smoothie, you can add more ice cubes or use a frozen banana instead of a fresh one. If you'd like a little extra sweetness, you could add a small amount of maple syrup or a low FODMAP sweetener like stevia. Just remember to account for this in your FODMAP count.

Overnight Chia Pudding with Kiwi and Pineapple

Preparation time: 10 minutes

Resting time: 8 hours (overnight)

Servings: 1-2

Ingredients:

- 1/4 cup (40 grams) chia seeds
- - 1 cup (240 mL) lactose-free milk or almond milk
- - 1 tablespoon (15 mL/21 grams) maple syrup
- - 1 small kiwi (about 70 grams), peeled and sliced
- - 1/2 cup (about 82.5 grams) pineapple chunks

Directions:

1. .In a glass or jar, mix together the chia seeds, milk, and maple syrup.
2. Stir well to make sure the chia seeds are evenly distributed and not clumping together.
3. Cover the glass or jar and place it in the refrigerator to set overnight (or for at least 8 hours).
4. In the morning, give the chia pudding a good stir to break up any clumps.
5. Top with the sliced kiwi and pineapple chunks.
6. Serve immediately, or cover and keep in the refrigerator for up to 3 days.

Nutrition: Calories: 350; Fat: 15g; Carbs: 45g; Protein: 10g

Notes and Variations: The consistency of chia pudding can be adjusted by adding more or less milk. If you prefer a looser pudding, add a bit more milk.

You can switch out the fruits based on your FODMAP tolerance levels. Other low FODMAP fruit options could include strawberries, oranges, or grapes. To increase the protein content, you could add a scoop of low FODMAP protein powder or some nuts or seeds. Always pay attention to portion sizes and adjust accordingly to keep it low FODMAP.

Almond Milk Smoothie with Strawberries and Banana

Preparation time: 5 minutes	Cooking time: 0 minutes	Servings: 1

Ingredients:

- 1/2 cup (75 grams) fresh strawberries
- - 1 cup (240 mL) unsweetened almond milk
- - A handful of ice cubes

Directions:

1. Add the banana, strawberries, almond milk, and ice cubes to a blender.
2. Blend until smooth and creamy.
3. Pour the smoothie into a glass and serve immediately.

Nutrition: Calories: 150; Fat: 4g; Carbs: 30g; Protein: 3g

Notes and Variations: You can add a scoop of low FODMAP protein powder to increase the protein content. You can replace the strawberries with other low FODMAP fruits like blueberries or raspberries, but always pay attention to portion sizes.

Lactose Free Yogurt with Cinnamon and Banana slices

Preparation time: 5 minutes	Cooking time: 0 minutes	Servings: 1

Ingredients:

- 1 cup lactose-free yogurt (240 grams)
- - 1 medium ripe banana (approximately 120 grams)
- - 1/2 teaspoon ground cinnamon (1.3 grams)
- - Optional: 1 teaspoon of chia seeds (4 grams) or a small handful of low FODMAP nuts like walnuts for added texture

Directions:

1. Peel and slice the banana.
2. In a bowl, stir the cinnamon into the lactose-free yogurt.
3. Arrange the banana slices on top of the yogurt.
4. If using, sprinkle the chia seeds or nuts on top of the banana slices.

Nutrition: Calories: 200; Fat: 2.5g; Carbs: 37g; Protein: 11g

Notes and Variations: To increase the protein content, you can add a scoop of low FODMAP protein powder to the yogurt. As bananas become higher in FODMAPs as they ripen, choose a banana that is ripe but not overripe. Always check the label of your lactose-free yogurt to ensure it doesn't contain any high FODMAP ingredients like inulin, honey, or high fructose corn syrup.

Tortilla Wrap with Scrambled Eggs and Cheddar Cheese

Preparation time: 5 minutes

Cooking time: 10 minutes

Servings: 1

Ingredients:

- - 2 medium-sized corn tortillas (about 50 grams)
- - 2 large eggs (about 100 grams)
- - 1 ounce cheddar cheese (about 28 grams)
- - 1 tablespoon olive oil (about 14 grams)
- - Salt and pepper to taste

Directions:

1. In a bowl, crack the eggs and whisk them until the yolks and whites are fully combined. Season with salt and pepper.
2. Heat the olive oil in a non-stick pan over medium heat.
3. Pour the beaten eggs into the pan and let them cook undisturbed for a few seconds until they start to set around the edges.
4. Stir the eggs constantly until they're mostly cooked but still slightly runny.
5. Sprinkle the cheddar cheese over the eggs and let it melt into them.
6. Warm the corn tortillas in a dry skillet over medium heat for about 30 seconds on each side.
7. Spoon the scrambled eggs onto the warm tortillas. Fold the tortilla over the eggs and serve immediately.

Nutrition: Calories: 450; Fat: 30g; Carbs: 24g; Protein: 20g

Notes and Variations: Feel free to add low FODMAP vegetables like bell peppers or spinach to your scrambled eggs for added nutrients. If you're lactose intolerant but can tolerate small amounts of lactose, you can use regular cheddar cheese. Hard cheeses like cheddar are low in lactose.

Buckwheat Porridge with Blueberries and Banana Slices

Preparation time: 10 minutes

Cooking time: 20 minutes

Servings: 2

Ingredients:

- 1/2 cup of raw buckwheat groats (about 85 grams)
- 2 cups of water (about 480 milliliters)
- 1 pinch of salt

- 1/2 cup of blueberries (about 75 grams)
- 1 medium banana (about 120 grams), sliced

Directions:

1. Rinse the buckwheat groats under cold water.
2. In a saucepan, bring the water to a boil.
3. Add the rinsed buckwheat and a pinch of salt to the boiling water.
4. Reduce the heat to low, cover, and simmer for about 20 minutes, or until the buckwheat is tender.
5. Once the buckwheat is cooked, remove from heat and let it sit covered for 10 minutes.
6. After the porridge has set, fluff it with a fork.
7. Serve the porridge in bowls topped with blueberries and banana slices.

Nutrition: Calories: 220; Fat: 2g; Carbs: 50g; Protein: 6g

Notes and Variations: If you want a creamier texture, you can cook the buckwheat in almond milk instead of water. You can also add a sprinkle of cinnamon or drizzle of maple syrup on top for added flavor.

Baked Frittata with Spinach and Tomatoes

Preparation time: 10 minutes

Cooking time: 20 minutes

Servings: 2

Ingredients:

- 4 large eggs
- 1/4 cup (about 60 milliliters) lactose-free milk
- Salt and pepper to taste
- 1 cup (about 30 grams) fresh spinach, chopped

- 1/2 cup (about 75 grams) cherry tomatoes, halved
- 1 tablespoon (about 15 milliliters) garlic-infused oil

Directions:

1. Preheat your oven to 375°F (190°C).
2. In a medium bowl, whisk together the eggs, lactose-free milk, salt, and pepper.
3. Heat the garlic-infused oil in an oven-safe skillet over medium heat.
4. Add the spinach to the skillet and cook until wilted, about 2-3 minutes.
5. Add the tomatoes to the skillet and cook for an additional minute.
6. Pour the egg mixture over the spinach and tomatoes, stirring gently to distribute the ingredients evenly.
7. Transfer the skillet to the preheated oven and bake for about 15-20 minutes, or until the eggs are set and slightly golden.
8. Remove from the oven and let it cool slightly before serving.

Nutrition: Calories: 210; Fat: 15g; Carbs: 4g; Protein: 14g

Notes and Variations: Feel free to add other low FODMAP vegetables or a bit of low FODMAP cheese like cheddar or feta. Always check your garlic-infused oil to make sure it doesn't contain any actual garlic pieces, as these can increase the FODMAP content.

Banana Buckwheat Pancakes

Preparation time: 15 minutes

Cooking time: 20 minutes

Servings: 2

Ingredients:

- 1 medium ripe banana
- 2 large eggs
- 1/2 cup (about 120 milliliters) almond milk
- 1 cup (about 120 grams) buckwheat flour
- 1 teaspoon (about 5 milliliters) vanilla extract
- 1/2 teaspoon (about 2.5 milliliters) baking powder
- A pinch of salt
- 1 tablespoon (about 15 milliliters) vegetable oil for cooking

Directions:

1. In a medium bowl, mash the ripe banana with a fork until smooth.
2. Add the eggs, almond milk, and vanilla extract to the bowl and mix until well combined.
3. In a separate bowl, combine the buckwheat flour, baking powder, and salt.
4. Gradually add the dry ingredients to the wet ingredients, mixing until just combined.
5. Heat the vegetable oil in a large non-stick skillet over medium heat.
6. Pour 1/4 cup (about 60 milliliters) of the pancake batter into the skillet for each pancake. Cook until bubbles form on the surface, then flip and cook until golden brown.
7. Serve the pancakes warm with your favorite low FODMAP toppings.

Nutrition: Calories: 370; Fat: 11g; Carbs: 58g; Protein: 14g

Notes and Variations: These pancakes are naturally sweet thanks to the ripe banana, but you can add a drizzle of maple syrup for extra sweetness if desired. Feel free to add a sprinkle of cinnamon or nutmeg to the batter for additional flavor.

Remember to use pure buckwheat flour as it is low in FODMAPs, while some other types of buckwheat products like soba noodles can be high in FODMAPs.

Buckwheat Crepes
with Banana and Maple Syrup

Preparation time: 15 minutes

Cooking time: 20 minutes

Servings: 2

Ingredients:

- 1 cup (about 120 grams) buckwheat flour
- 2 large eggs
- 1 1/2 cups (about 355 milliliters) almond milk
- A pinch of salt

- 1 tablespoon (about 15 milliliters) vegetable oil for cooking
- 2 medium bananas, sliced
- Maple syrup for serving

Directions:

1. In a large bowl, whisk together the buckwheat flour, eggs, almond milk, and salt until smooth.
2. Heat a small amount of the vegetable oil in a non-stick skillet over medium heat.
3. Pour about 1/4 cup (about 60 milliliters) of the batter into the skillet and tilt the pan to spread the batter evenly.
4. Cook the crepe for about 2 minutes, or until the bottom is light golden brown. Flip and cook the other side for 1 minute.
5. Repeat with the remaining batter.
6. Fill each crepe with banana slices and roll up. Drizzle with maple syrup before serving.

Nutrition: Calories: 500; Fat: 12g; Carbs: 90g; Protein: 14g

Notes and Variations: These crepes can be filled with your favorite low FODMAP fruits if bananas aren't to your liking. Instead of maple syrup, you can also drizzle a bit of melted dark chocolate on top for a different flavor profile.

Lactose-Free Yogurt Parfait

Preparation time: 10 minutes

Cooking time: 0 minutes

Servings: 1

Ingredients:

- 1 cup (about 225 grams) lactose-free yogurt
- 1/2 cup (about 50 grams) gluten-free granola
- 1/2 cup (about 75 grams) strawberries, hulled and sliced
- 1 tablespoon (about 15 milliliters) maple syrup (optional)

Directions:

1. In a glass or jar, layer half of the yogurt at the bottom.
2. Next, layer half of the granola, followed by half of the strawberries.
3. Repeat these layers with the remaining yogurt, granola, and strawberries.
4. Drizzle with maple syrup if you prefer a bit of extra sweetness.
5. Serve immediately, or refrigerate until ready to eat.

Nutrition: Calories: 350; Fat: 12g; Carbs: 45g; Protein: 15g

Notes and Variations: You can customize your parfait with different types of berries or fruits that are low in FODMAPs. The granola can be replaced with other low FODMAP cereals if you prefer. Honey can be used instead of maple syrup but be mindful of the portion to keep it within low FODMAP guidelines.

Scrambled Tofu

Preparation time: 5 minutes

Cooking time: 10 minutes

Servings: 1

Ingredients:

- 1/2 block (about 200 grams) firm tofu
- 1 tablespoon (about 15 milliliters) garlic-infused oil
- 1/4 teaspoon (about 1 gram) turmeric
- 1/4 teaspoon (about 1 gram) paprika
- Salt and pepper to taste
- 1 slice of gluten-free bread (to serve)

Directions:

1. Drain the tofu and crumble it into small pieces.
2. Heat the garlic-infused oil in a pan over medium heat.
3. Add the crumbled tofu to the pan.
4. Season with turmeric, paprika, salt, and pepper.
5. Stir well to combine the spices with the tofu and cook for about 10 minutes, or until the tofu is heated through and starting to get a bit crispy.
6. Serve the scrambled tofu on a slice of gluten-free bread.

Nutrition: Calories: 325; Fat: 16g; Carbs: 25g; Protein: 22g

Notes and Variations: You can add other low FODMAP vegetables to the scramble, like spinach or bell peppers, for additional nutrition and flavor. You can also use this scrambled tofu as a filling for a low FODMAP tortilla wrap or as a topping for a salad.

Banana and Coconut Pancakes

Preparation time: 10 minutes   Cooking time: 15 minutes   Servings: 2

Ingredients:

- 1 ripe banana (about 120 grams)
- 2 large eggs
- 1/2 cup (about 50 grams) coconut flour
- 1/4 cup (about 60 milliliters) unsweetened almond milk
- 1/2 teaspoon (about 2.5 grams) baking powder
- Pinch of salt
- 1-2 teaspoons (about 5-10 milliliters) coconut oil, for cooking
- Maple syrup, for serving (optional)

Directions:

1. Mash the ripe banana in a bowl until it's free of large lumps.
2. Crack the eggs into the bowl with the banana and whisk together.
3. Add the coconut flour, almond milk, baking powder, and salt. Mix until you have a uniform batter.
4. Heat a non-stick skillet over medium heat and add a bit of coconut oil.
5. Spoon batter onto the skillet to form pancakes of your desired size.
6. Cook for about 2-3 minutes on each side, or until golden brown.
7. Serve hot, with a drizzle of maple syrup if desired.

Nutrition: Calories: 300; Fat: 16g; Carbs: 32g; Protein: 10g

Notes and Variations: Be sure to keep the heat on medium to avoid burning the pancakes, as coconut flour can burn faster than regular flour. You can top these pancakes with a small amount of low FODMAP fruits like strawberries or blueberries for extra flavor and nutrition.

LUNCH RECIPES

Grilled Chicken Salad

Preparation time: 15 minutes

Cooking time: 10 minutes

Servings: 1-2

Ingredients:

- 1 chicken breast (approximately 100-150g)
- Mixed salad greens (2 cups or approximately 60g)
- 2 medium tomatoes (approximately 200g)
- Olive oil (2 tablespoons or approximately 30ml)
- Balsamic vinegar (1 tablespoon or approximately 15ml)
- -Salt and pepper to taste

Directions:

1. Preheat the grill on medium heat.
2. Rub the chicken breast with 1 tablespoon of olive oil, and season it with salt and pepper.
3. Grill the chicken breast for about 5 minutes on each side, or until it's fully cooked and no longer pink in the center.
4. While the chicken is grilling, wash the mixed greens and tomatoes. Slice the tomatoes into quarters or smaller slices based on your preference.
5. Toss the mixed greens and tomatoes in a bowl. Drizzle with the remaining olive oil and balsamic vinegar, and season with a little salt and pepper.
6. When the chicken is done, let it rest for a few minutes, then slice it into thin strips.
7. Place the grilled chicken strips on top of the salad and serve immediately. Enjoy!

Nutrition: Calories: 265; Fat: 15g; Carbs: 10g; Protein: 25g

Notes and Variations: You can customize this recipe by adding other low-FODMAP veggies like cucumbers or bell peppers. If you're vegetarian, you can replace the chicken with tofu or tempeh.

Rice Noodles with Shrimp

Preparation time: 20 minutes

Cooking time: 15 minutes

Servings: 1-2

Ingredients:

- Rice noodles (2 ounces or approximately 57g)
- 10 medium-sized shrimp, peeled and deveined (approximately 150g)
- 1 medium bell pepper, sliced (approximately 120g)
- Garlic-infused olive oil (1 tablespoon or approximately 15ml)
- Low-sodium soy sauce (2 tablespoons or approximately 30ml)
- Salt and pepper to taste

Directions:

1. Cook the rice noodles according to the package instructions. Once cooked, drain and set aside.
2. While the noodles are cooking, heat the garlic-infused olive oil in a skillet over medium heat.
3. Add the shrimp to the skillet and cook until they turn pink, about 2-3 minutes per side.
4. Add the sliced bell peppers to the skillet and stir-fry until they're tender-crisp, about 2-3 minutes.
5. Add the cooked noodles to the skillet, and pour the soy sauce over the top. Toss everything together to combine, and season with salt and pepper.
6. Cook for another 2-3 minutes until everything is heated through, then serve immediately. Enjoy!

Nutrition: Calories: 320; Fat: 7g; Carbs: 45g; Protein: 20g

Notes and Variations: You can replace the shrimp with tofu or chicken for a different protein option. Adjust cooking time accordingly. Be sure to use garlic-infused oil that doesn't contain actual garlic pieces, as these can increase FODMAP content.

Gluten-Free Turkey Wrap

Preparation time: 10 minutes

Cooking time: 0 minutes

Servings: 1-2

Ingredients:

- Gluten-free tortilla (1 piece or about 40-60g, depending on brand)
- Turkey slices (4 ounces or about 113g)
- Lettuce leaves, rinsed and dried (1 cup or about 50g)
- 1 medium tomato, sliced (approximately 180g)
- Mayonnaise, suitable for the FODMAP diet (1 tablespoon or about 15g)
- Salt and pepper to taste

Directions:

1. Spread the mayonnaise evenly across the gluten-free tortilla.
2. Layer the turkey slices on top of the mayo, leaving a small border around the edge of the tortilla.
3. Arrange the lettuce leaves on top of the turkey, followed by the tomato slices.
4. Sprinkle a little salt and pepper over the tomato.
5. Roll up the tortilla tightly, starting from one side and working your way to the other.
6. Cut the wrap in half, if desired, and serve immediately. Enjoy this refreshing and easy-to-make meal!

Nutrition: Calories: 400; Fat: 15g; Carbs: 35g; Protein: 30g

Notes and Variations: You can replace the turkey with other low-FODMAP meats like chicken or ham. Add a slice of lactose-free cheese for additional flavor, if tolerated. If you prefer a warm meal, you can heat the wrap in a pan or sandwich press until it's crispy and heated through. Just be sure to use a gluten-free tortilla that can withstand heat.

Quinoa Salad

Preparation time: 15 minutes

Cooking time: 20 minutes

Servings: 1-2

Ingredients:

- Quinoa (1/2 cup or about 85g)
- - Water (1 cup or about 240ml)
- - Diced cucumber (1/2 cup or about 75g)
- - Cherry tomatoes, halved (1/2 cup or about 75g)
- - Lemon juice (2 tablespoons or about 30ml)
- - Olive oil (1 tablespoon or about 15ml)
- - Salt and pepper to taste
- - Fresh parsley, chopped (optional)

Directions:

1. . Rinse the quinoa under cold water until the water runs clear. This helps remove the quinoa's natural coating, which can make it taste bitter or soapy.
2. In a small saucepan, bring the water to a boil. Add the rinsed quinoa, reduce the heat to low, cover, and simmer for about 15 minutes, or until the quinoa has absorbed all the water and is fluffy.
3. While the quinoa is cooling, prepare your vegetables. Dice the cucumber and halve the cherry tomatoes.
4. In a large bowl, combine the cooked and cooled quinoa, cucumber, and tomatoes.
5. Drizzle with olive oil and lemon juice, season with salt and pepper, and toss until everything is well combined.
6. If desired, garnish with fresh parsley before serving.

Nutrition: Calories: 310; Fat: 12g; Carbs: 42g; Protein: 11g

Notes and Variations: You can add other low-FODMAP vegetables like bell peppers or radishes for extra crunch. For a protein boost, consider adding grilled chicken or canned tuna.

Tuna Salad

Preparation time: 10 minutes

Cooking time: 0 minutes

Servings: 1-2

Ingredients:

- Canned tuna in water, drained (1 can or about 140g)
- Diced celery (1/2 cup or about 60g)
- Diced carrots (1/2 cup or about 60g)
- Low-FODMAP mayonnaise (2 tablespoons or about 30ml)
- Salt and pepper to taste
- Lemon juice (optional)

Directions:

1. Open the can of tuna, drain the water, and put the tuna in a mixing bowl.
2. Wash and dice the celery and carrots into small pieces.
3. Add the diced vegetables to the bowl with the tuna.
4. Add the mayonnaise to the bowl and stir until everything is well combined. If the salad seems too dry, you can add a bit more mayonnaise.
5. Season with salt and pepper to taste. If desired, add a squeeze of lemon juice for extra tanginess.
6. Serve the tuna salad on its own, or use it as a filling for sandwiches or wraps.

Nutrition: Calories: 200; Fat: 11g; Carbs: 6g; Protein: 20g

Notes and Variations: You can add other low-FODMAP vegetables like cucumber or bell peppers for extra crunch. For a dairy-free option, use a dairy-free mayonnaise substitute. For a different flavor profile, try adding herbs like dill or parsley.

Baked Sweet Potato

Preparation time: 10 minutes

Cooking time: 45 minutes

Servings: 1-2

Ingredients:

- Medium sweet potato (1 or about 130g)
- Lactose-free Greek yogurt (2 tablespoons or about 30ml)
- Chopped fresh chives (1 tablespoon or about 15ml)
- Olive oil (1 teaspoon or about 5ml)
- Salt and pepper to taste

Directions:

1. Preheat your oven to 425°F (220°C).
2. Wash the sweet potato and pat it dry. Using a fork, poke holes all over the sweet potato. This helps steam to escape during the baking process.
3. Lightly coat the sweet potato in olive oil, then season with salt and pepper.

4. Place the sweet potato on a baking sheet and bake for about 45 minutes, or until it is easily pierced with a fork.
5. Once the sweet potato is done, let it cool for a few minutes before cutting it open.
6. Top the sweet potato with the lactose-free Greek yogurt and chopped chives.
7. Serve immediately and enjoy your healthy and delicious low-FODMAP meal!

Nutrition: Calories: 180; Fat: 1.5g; Carbs: 40g; Protein: 4g

Notes and Variations: For added protein, you can top your sweet potato with cooked chicken or turkey. You can use other low-FODMAP herbs like parsley or dill in place of the chives. If you're not a fan of Greek yogurt, you can top your sweet potato with a lactose-free sour cream instead.

Caprese Salad

Preparation time: 15 minutes

Cooking time: 0 minutes

Servings: 1-2

Ingredients:

- Fresh mozzarella (4 oz or about 113g)
- Ripe tomatoes (2 medium-sized or about 280g)
- Fresh basil leaves (10-12 leaves)
- Balsamic reduction (1 tablespoon or about 15ml)
- Extra virgin olive oil (1 tablespoon or about 15ml)
- Salt and pepper to taste

Directions:

1. Slice the fresh mozzarella and ripe tomatoes into evenly thick slices.
2. Arrange the mozzarella, tomatoes, and fresh basil leaves on a plate, alternating and overlapping them for a nice presentation.
3. Drizzle the salad with the balsamic reduction and extra virgin olive oil.
4. Season with salt and pepper to taste.
5. Serve immediately and enjoy this light, fresh, and low-FODMAP Caprese Salad!

Nutrition: Calories: 250; Fat: 18g; Carbs: 10g; Protein: 14g

Notes and Variations: Make sure to choose a low-FODMAP balsamic reduction, as some varieties can contain high-FODMAP ingredients like garlic or onion. If you want to add more protein to this salad, you can top it with grilled chicken or shrimp.

Egg Salad

Preparation time: 15 minutes

Cooking time: 0 minutes

Servings: 1-2

Ingredients:

- Boiled eggs (4 medium or about 200g)
- Mayonnaise (2 tablespoons or about 30ml)
- Mustard (1 teaspoon or about 5ml)
- Scallions, green parts only (2 tablespoons, finely chopped or about 15g)
- Salt and pepper to taste

Directions:

1. Peel and chop the boiled eggs into small pieces.
2. In a bowl, mix together the mayonnaise and mustard until well combined.
3. Add the chopped eggs and scallions to the bowl, and gently stir until everything is evenly coated in the mayonnaise-mustard mixture.
4. Season with salt and pepper to taste.
5. You can serve this egg salad immediately, or cover it and refrigerate for later. It makes a delicious filling for sandwiches, or you can serve it on lettuce leaves for a low-carb option.

Nutrition: Calories: 310; Fat: 26g; Carbs: 2g; Protein: 18g

Notes and Variations: To add some crunch to your egg salad, try adding some chopped celery or bell pepper. Make sure to use a low-FODMAP mayonnaise, as some varieties can contain high-FODMAP ingredients like garlic or onion.

Rice Paper Rolls with Shrimp

Preparation time: 30 minutes

Cooking time: 10 minutes

Servings: 1-2

Ingredients:

- Rice paper sheets (4 or about 40g)
- Cooked shrimp (100g or 3.5oz)
- Carrot (1 medium or about 60g), julienned
- Cucumber (half or about 100g), julienned
- Fresh mint leaves (10 leaves or about 5g)

For the dipping sauce**:
- - Rice vinegar (1 tablespoon or about 15ml)
- - Soy sauce (1 tablespoon or about 15ml)
- - A pinch of sugar

Directions:

1. Prepare your ingredients: cook the shrimp if not pre-cooked, and julienne the carrot and cucumber.
2. Soak each rice paper sheet in warm water until it becomes soft and pliable, then lay it flat on a clean surface.

3. Place a few mint leaves on the rice paper, followed by some of the shrimp, carrot, and cucumber.
4. Fold the sides of the rice paper in, then roll it up tightly like a burrito. Repeat with the remaining rice paper sheets and fillings.
5. For the dipping sauce, mix together the rice vinegar, soy sauce, and sugar until the sugar is dissolved.
6. Serve the rice paper rolls with the dipping sauce on the side.

Nutrition: Calories: 250; Fat: 4g; Carbs: 30g; Protein: 20g

Notes and Variations: You can vary the fillings for the rice paper rolls depending on your tastes and what you have available. Other options could include bell pepper, lettuce, or cooked chicken. If you're not a fan of shrimp, you could substitute it with cooked chicken or tofu.

Zucchini Noodles with Garlic-infused Oil and Cherry Tomatoes

Preparation time: 15 minutes

Cooking time: 10 minutes

Servings: 1-2

Ingredients:

- Zucchinis (2 medium or about 500g), spiralized
- Garlic-infused olive oil (2 tablespoons or about 30ml)
- Cherry tomatoes (1 cup or about 150g), halved
- Salt and pepper to taste
- Fresh basil leaves for garnish

Directions:

1. Use a spiralizer to turn your zucchinis into noodles. If you don't have a spiralizer, you can use a vegetable peeler to create long, thin ribbons.
2. Heat the garlic-infused olive oil in a large skillet over medium heat.
3. Add the cherry tomatoes to the skillet and cook for 2-3 minutes, until they start to soften.
4. Add the zucchini noodles to the skillet, tossing them in the oil and tomatoes. Cook for another 2-3 minutes, until the noodles are tender but still have a bit of bite.
5. Season with salt and pepper to taste, then remove from the heat.
6. Serve the noodles garnished with fresh basil leaves.

Nutrition: Calories: 200; Fat: 13g; Carbs: 20g; Protein: 5g

Notes and Variations: You can add some grilled chicken or shrimp to this dish for extra protein. If you don't have cherry tomatoes, you can substitute them with any other type of tomato. Just make sure to chop them into small pieces. To make this dish even more flavorful, consider adding a sprinkle of Parmesan cheese on top. Just be aware that cheese can be high in lactose, so use it in moderation if you're sensitive.

Grilled Shrimp Salad with Lemon Dressing

Preparation time: 20 minutes	Cooking time: 10 minutes	Servings: 1-2

Ingredients:

- Shrimp (1/2 pound or about 225g), peeled and deveined
- Mixed salad greens (2 cups or about 60g)
- Cherry tomatoes (1/2 cup or about 75g), halved
- Cucumber (1/2 medium or about 150g), sliced

- Olive oil (1 tablespoon or about 15ml), for grilling
- Salt and pepper to taste
  For the Lemon Dressing
- Freshly squeezed lemon juice (2 tablespoons or about 30ml)
- Olive oil (2 tablespoons or about 30ml)
- Salt and pepper to taste

Directions:

1. Preheat your grill or grill pan over medium-high heat.
2. Toss the shrimp in the olive oil and season with salt and pepper.
3. Grill the shrimp for about 2-3 minutes on each side, until they are pink and cooked through.
4. While the shrimp are grilling, prepare the lemon dressing by whisking together the lemon juice, olive oil, salt, and pepper.
5. In a large bowl, combine the mixed salad greens, cherry tomatoes, and cucumber.
6. Add the grilled shrimp to the salad, then drizzle with the lemon dressing. Toss everything together until well combined.

Nutrition: Calories: 300; Fat: 18g; Carbs: 10g; Protein: 25g

Notes and Variations: For an added crunch, consider topping your salad with some toasted almond slices or sunflower seeds. You can also add other low-FODMAP vegetables to this salad, like bell peppers or radishes. If you're not a fan of shrimp, you can substitute it with grilled chicken or tofu.

Grilled Chicken Caesar Salad (without Garlic)

Preparation time: 15 minutes	Cooking time: 20 minutes	Servings: 1-2

Ingredients:

- Chicken breast (1 medium-sized or about 200g), boneless, skinless
- Romaine lettuce (2 cups or 474ml), chopped
- Parmesan cheese (1/4 cup or about 25g), shaved
- Olive oil (2 tablespoons or about 30ml)
- Lemon juice (1 tablespoon or about 15ml)
- Dijon mustard (1/2 teaspoon or about 2.5g)
- Worcestershire sauce (1/2 teaspoon or about 2.5ml)
- Salt and pepper to taste

Directions:

1. Preheat your grill or grill pan over medium heat.
2. Season the chicken breast with salt and pepper, then grill until cooked through, about 7 minutes per side. Let it rest for a few minutes, then slice.
3. In a large salad bowl, combine the chopped romaine lettuce and sliced chicken.
4. In a small bowl, whisk together the olive oil, lemon juice, Dijon mustard, Worcestershire sauce, salt, and pepper.
5. Drizzle the dressing over the salad and toss to combine. Top with shaved Parmesan cheese.

Nutrition: Calories: 375; Fat: 23g; Carbs: 4g; Protein: 37g

Notes and Variations: Traditional Caesar salads contain garlic and anchovies, both of which are high in FODMAPs.

Low-FODMAP Minestrone Soup

Preparation time: 15 minutes

Cooking time: 30 minutes

Servings: 1-2

Ingredients:

- Olive oil (1 tablespoon or about 15ml)
- Carrots (1/2 cup or about 65g), diced
- Red bell pepper (1/2 cup or about 75g), diced
- Zucchini (1/2 cup or about 90g), diced
- Green beans (1/2 cup or about 75g), cut into 1-inch pieces
- Canned diced tomatoes (1 cup or about 240g), no added onion or garlic
- Low-FODMAP vegetable broth (4 cups or about 1 liter)
- Quinoa (1/4 cup or about 45g), rinsed
- Salt and pepper to taste
- Fresh basil (1/4 cup or about 5g), for garnish

Directions:

1. Heat the olive oil in a large pot over medium heat.

2. Add the carrots, bell pepper, zucchini, and green beans to the pot. Cook, stirring occasionally, until the vegetables are softened (about 10 minutes).
3. Add the diced tomatoes and vegetable broth to the pot and bring to a simmer.
4. Stir in the quinoa and season with salt and pepper. Reduce the heat to low, cover the pot, and simmer for about 15 minutes, or until the quinoa is cooked.
5. Ladle the soup into bowls and garnish with fresh basil. Serve hot.

Nutrition: Calories: 210; Fat: 5g; Carbs: 38g; Protein: 6g

Notes and Variations: For a heartier soup, you can add cooked chicken or turkey. You can use other low-FODMAP vegetables if desired. Just be mindful of portion sizes to keep the dish low-FODMAP.

Baked Salmon with Lemon and Dill

Preparation time: 10 minutes

Cooking time: 20 minutes

Servings: 1-2

Ingredients:

- Fresh salmon fillet (6 ounces or about 170g)
- Salt and pepper to taste
- Fresh lemon slices (2-3 slices)
- Fresh dill (1 tablespoon or about 2g), chopped
- Olive oil (1 tablespoon or about 15ml)

Directions:
1. Preheat your oven to 400 degrees Fahrenheit (about 200 degrees Celsius).
2. Pat the salmon dry and season with salt and pepper on both sides.
3. Place the salmon on a piece of aluminum foil large enough to fold over and seal.
4. Top the salmon with the lemon slices and dill, then drizzle the olive oil over the top.
5. Fold the sides of the foil over the salmon to cover and completely seal the packet closed.
6. Bake in the preheated oven for 15-20 minutes, or until the salmon flakes easily with a fork.

Nutrition: Calories: 365; Fat: 25g; Carbs: 0g; Protein: 34g

Notes and Variations: For a complete meal, serve the salmon with a side of steamed low-FODMAP vegetables or a green salad. Be sure to remove the skin from the salmon fillet to reduce the fat content if desired. Fresh rosemary or thyme can be used in place of dill for a different flavor profile.

Greek Salad with Olives and Feta

Preparation time: 15 minutes

Cooking time: 0 minutes

Servings: 1-2

Ingredients:

- Lettuce (2 cups or 473ml), chopped
- Cherry tomatoes (1 cup or 150g), halved
- Cucumber (1 medium or about 150g), diced
- Red bell pepper (1 medium or about 119g), diced
- Olives (10 or about 40g), pitted and halved
- Feta cheese (1/4 cup or about 28g), crumbled
- - Olive oil (1 tablespoon or about 15ml)
- - Red wine vinegar (1 tablespoon or about 15ml)
- Dried oregano (1/2 teaspoon or about 1g)
- Salt and pepper to taste

Directions:

1. In a large salad bowl, combine the lettuce, cherry tomatoes, cucumber, bell pepper, olives, and feta cheese.
2. In a small bowl, whisk together the olive oil, red wine vinegar, dried oregano, salt, and pepper.
3. Drizzle the dressing over the salad and toss gently to combine.

Nutrition: Calories: 202; Fat: 16g; Carbs: 9g; Protein: 5g

Notes and Variations: For added protein, consider adding grilled chicken or shrimp. For a lower-sodium option, reduce the amount of olives and feta cheese.

Turkey Wrap with Gluten-Free Tortilla, Lettuce and Tomato

Preparation time: 10 minutes	Cooking time: 0 minutes	Servings: 1

Ingredients:

- Gluten-free tortilla (1 piece or about 45g)
- Turkey slices (3 ounces or about 85g), cooked
- Romaine lettuce (1 cup or about 237ml), shredded
- Tomato (1 medium or about 123g), sliced
- Mayonnaise (1 tablespoon or about 15g), low-FODMAP
- Salt and pepper to taste

Directions:

1. Lay out the gluten-free tortilla on a flat surface.
2. Spread the mayonnaise over one side of the tortilla.
3. Lay the turkey slices over the mayonnaise.
4. Add the shredded lettuce and tomato slices on top of the turkey.
5. Season with salt and pepper.
6. Roll up the tortilla tightly, tucking in the sides as you go.
7. Slice the wrap in half diagonally and serve.

Nutrition: Calories: 310; Fat: 12g; Carbs: 30g; Protein: 18g

Notes and Variations: Make sure your turkey slices are low-FODMAP. For a bit of extra flavor, consider adding a slice of Swiss or cheddar cheese. If you're vegetarian, you can replace the turkey with tofu or tempeh. Just make sure they're plain and not marinated in high-FODMAP sauces.

Gluten-Free Pasta Salad with Cherry Tomatoes and Olives

Preparation time: 15 minutes	Cooking time: 10 minutes	Servings: 2

Ingredients:

- Gluten-free pasta (1 cup or about 140g dry)
- Cherry tomatoes (1 cup or about 150g), halved
- Black olives (1/4 cup or about 30g), pitted and sliced
- Feta cheese (1/4 cup or about 35g), crumbled
- Olive oil (2 tablespoons or about 30ml)
- Lemon juice (1 tablespoon or about 15ml)
- Fresh basil leaves (a handful), torn
- Salt and pepper to taste

Directions:

1. Cook the pasta according to the package instructions. Once done, drain and rinse under cold water to cool. Set aside.
2. In a large bowl, combine the halved cherry tomatoes, sliced black olives, and crumbled feta cheese.
3. Add the cooled pasta to the bowl and mix well.
4. In a small bowl, whisk together the olive oil and lemon juice. Season with salt and pepper.
5. Pour the dressing over the pasta salad and toss until everything is well coated.
6. Sprinkle the torn basil leaves over the top and give the salad one final mix.
7. Serve immediately, or refrigerate for an hour to let the flavors meld together.

Nutrition: Calories: 400; Fat: 16g; Carbs: 55g; Protein: 10g

Notes and Variations: You can add in other low-FODMAP vegetables like cucumber or bell pepper for extra crunch. For a protein boost, consider adding cooked chicken or shrimp.

Brown Rice Salad with Roasted Vegetables-

Preparation time: 15 minutes	Cooking time: 45 minutes	Servings: 1-2

Ingredients:

- 1 cup (185 grams) brown rice
- 2 cups (500 mL) water
- Salt to taste
- 2 bell peppers (any color), cut into chunks
- 1 medium zucchini, cut into half-moons
- 2 tablespoons (30 mL) olive oil
- 1 tablespoon (15 mL) balsamic vinegar
- 1/2 teaspoon (2.5 grams) dried basil
- 1/2 teaspoon (2.5 grams) dried oregano
- Black pepper to taste
- 1 tablespoon (15 mL) lemon juice
- 1 tablespoon (15 mL) extra virgin olive oil
- 2 tablespoons (6 grams) fresh chives, chopped

Directions:

1. Preheat your oven to 400°F (200°C).
2. In a saucepan, bring the water to a boil. Add the brown rice and a pinch of salt, then reduce the heat to low, cover the pot, and let it simmer for 45 minutes, or until the rice is tender and all the water is absorbed.
3. While the rice is cooking, toss the bell peppers and zucchini with the olive oil, balsamic vinegar, basil, oregano, salt, and black pepper. Spread them out on a baking sheet and roast in the preheated oven for about 20 minutes, or until they are tender and starting to brown.
4. Once the vegetables and rice are done, let them cool for a few minutes. Then combine them in a large bowl, adding the lemon juice, extra virgin olive oil, and chives. Toss well to combine.
5. Taste and adjust the seasoning if needed. You can serve this salad warm, at room temperature, or chilled.

Nutrition: Calories: 350; Fat: 12g; Carbs: 56g; Protein: 7g

Notes and Variations: Feel free to vary the vegetables based on what you have on hand and what's in season. Other low FODMAP options include carrots, eggplant, and butternut squash. For added protein, you could toss in some grilled chicken, tofu, or canned lentils (make sure to stick to a safe serving size of lentils to keep it low FODMAP).

Lentil Soup with Carrots and Cumin

Preparation time: 10 minutes

Cooking time: 45 minutes

Servings: 1-2

Ingredients:

- 1/2 cup (100 grams) dried green lentils
- 2 cups (500 mL) water
- 1/2 tablespoon (7 mL) olive oil
- 1 medium carrot, diced
- 1/4 teaspoon (1 gram) cumin
- Salt and black pepper to taste
- 2 tablespoons (6 grams) fresh parsley, chopped

Directions:

1. Put the lentils under cold running water until the water runs clear.
2. In a large pot, combine the lentils and water. Bring to a boil over high heat, then reduce the heat to low, cover the pot, and let it simmer for about 30 minutes, or until the lentils are tender.
3. Meanwhile, heat the olive oil in a skillet over medium heat. Add the diced carrot and cook for about 5 minutes, or until it starts to soften.
4. Stir in the cumin and cook for another minute, then remove from the heat.
5. Once the lentils are done, add the cooked carrot and cumin to the pot. Season with salt and black pepper to taste.
6. Using an immersion blender, blend the soup until it reaches your desired consistency. If you prefer a chunkier soup, you can skip this step or only partially blend it.
7. Ladle the soup into bowls, sprinkle with the chopped parsley, and serve.

Nutrition: Calories: 200; Fat: 3g; Carbs: 30g; Protein: 14g

Notes and Variations: Keep in mind that while lentils are generally considered low FODMAP, they can become high FODMAP in larger servings. If you're sensitive to them, you might want to start with a smaller serving of this soup and see how you tolerate it. For extra flavor, you could add a bay leaf or a couple of cloves of garlic (which are low FODMAP when used as an infusion) to the pot along with the lentils and water, then remove them before blending the soup.

Baked Tilapia with Lemon and Dill

Preparation time: 10 minutes

Cooking time: 20 minutes

Servings: 1-2

Ingredients:

- 2 tilapia fillets (about 4-6 ounces or 113-170 grams each)
- 1 tablespoon (15 mL) olive oil
- Salt and black pepper to taste
- 1 lemon (use both for zest and juice)
- 1 tablespoon (1 gram) fresh dill, chopped
- Lemon slices and additional dill for garnish (optional)

Directions:

1. Preheat your oven to 400°F (200°C) and line a baking sheet with parchment paper.
2. Place the tilapia fillets on the prepared baking sheet and drizzle with olive oil. Season with salt and black pepper to taste.
3. Zest the lemon and sprinkle the zest over the tilapia. Then cut the lemon in half and squeeze the juice of one half over the fillets.
4. Sprinkle the chopped dill over the tilapia.
5. Bake for 15-20 minutes, or until the fish flakes easily with a fork.

6. Remove from the oven and garnish with lemon slices and additional dill, if desired. Serve immediately.

Nutrition: Calories: 180; Fat: 4g; Carbs: 34g; Protein: 1g

Notes and Variations: While this recipe calls for tilapia, you could easily substitute another type of white fish if you prefer. If you're not a fan of dill, feel free to use another herb. Parsley or basil would both work well.

Riced Noodles with Peanut Sauce

Preparation time: 10 minutes

Cooking time: 10 minutes

Servings: 2

Ingredients:

- 4 ounces (113 grams) rice noodles
- 2 tablespoons (30 milliliters) peanut butter
- 1 tablespoon (15 milliliters) soy sauce (ensure it's gluten-free for Low FODMAP)
- 1 tablespoon (15 milliliters) maple syrup

- 1/4 cup (60 milliliters) water
- 1 tablespoon (15 milliliters) garlic-infused oil
- 1 cup (about 90 grams) diced bell pepper
- 1 cup (about 128 grams) diced zucchini
- Optional: 1 green onion (green part only), sliced for garnish

Directions:

1. Cook the rice noodles according to the package instructions. Drain and set aside.
2. In a small bowl, whisk together the peanut butter, soy sauce, maple syrup, and water until smooth.
3. Heat the garlic-infused oil in a skillet over medium heat. Add the bell pepper and zucchini, and sauté until tender.
4. Add the cooked noodles to the skillet with the vegetables, then pour the peanut sauce over the top. Stir to combine.
5. Serve the noodles hot, garnished with sliced green onion if desired.

Nutrition: Calories: 385; Fat: 14g; Carbs: 57g; Protein: 10g

Notes and Variations: You can add cooked shrimp or chicken for extra protein. Be sure to adjust the nutritional information accordingly. The zucchini and bell pepper can be swapped out for other low FODMAP veggies like carrots and eggplant.

Veggie Tacos

Preparation time: 15 minutes

Cooking time: 15 minutes

Servings: 2

Ingredients:

- 4 small corn tortillas
- - 1 cup (about 149 grams) diced bell pepper
- - 1 cup (about 124 grams) diced zucchini
- - 1 tablespoon (15 milliliters) garlic-infused oil
- - 1/2 cup (about 56 grams) cheddar cheese, shredded
- - Salt and pepper to taste
- - Optional: fresh cilantro and lime wedges for garnish

Directions:

1. Heat the garlic-infused oil in a skillet over medium heat. Add the bell pepper and zucchini, season with salt and pepper, and sauté until tender.
2. Warm the tortillas in a dry skillet over medium heat until they are soft and pliable.
3. Distribute the sautéed vegetables evenly among the tortillas and sprinkle with cheddar cheese.
4. Fold each tortilla in half and return to the skillet. Cook each side until the cheese is melted and the tortilla is crispy.
5. Serve the tacos hot, garnished with fresh cilantro and lime wedges if desired.

Nutrition: Calories: 362; Fat: 18g; Carbs: 38g; Protein: 13g

Notes and Variations: You can add cooked chicken or beef for extra protein but be sure to adjust the nutritional information accordingly.

Quinoa Salad

Preparation time: 10 minutes	Cooking time: 20 minutes	Servings: 2

Ingredients:

- 1/2 cup (about 90 grams) uncooked quinoa
- 1 cup (about 250 milliliters) water
- 1/2 cup (about 75 grams) diced cucumber
- 1/2 cup (about 75 grams) halved cherry tomatoes
- 1/4 cup (about 4 grams) fresh chopped herbs (parsley, chives, etc.)
- Juice of 1/2 a lemon
- 2 tablespoons (about 30 milliliters) extra virgin olive oil
- Salt and pepper to taste

Directions:

1. Rinse the quinoa under cold water until the water runs clear.
2. In a pot, bring the water to a boil. Add the quinoa, reduce the heat to low, cover, and let it simmer for 15-20 minutes until the water is absorbed and the quinoa is fluffy.
3. Let the quinoa cool completely.
4. In a large bowl, combine the cooled quinoa, cucumber, cherry tomatoes, and fresh herbs.

5. Drizzle with lemon juice and olive oil, and season with salt and pepper to taste. Toss to combine.
6. Serve immediately, or refrigerate until ready to serve.

Nutrition: Calories: 303; Fat: 15g; Carbs: 37g; Protein: 7g

Notes and Variations: You can add lower FODMAP vegetables or even some cooked chicken or tofu for extra protein.

Stir-Fried Shrimp with Bell Peppers

Preparation time: 15 minutes

Cooking time: 15 minutes

Servings: 2

Ingredients:

- 1/2 pound (about 225 grams) fresh shrimp, peeled and deveined
- 1 medium-size red bell pepper (about 150 grams), thinly sliced
- 1 tablespoon (about 15 milliliters) garlic-infused olive oil
- 1 tablespoon (about 15 milliliters) gluten-free soy sauce or tamari
- Salt and pepper to taste

Directions:

1. Heat the garlic-infused olive oil in a large skillet or wok over medium-high heat.
2. Add the thinly sliced bell pepper to the pan and stir-fry for about 5 minutes until they are tender.
3. Add the shrimp, soy sauce, and a pinch of salt and pepper. Continue to stir-fry for another 5-7 minutes or until the shrimp is cooked through.
4. Serve the stir-fry over cooked rice or quinoa, if desired.

Nutrition: Calories: 176; Fat: 5g; Carbs: 7g; Protein: 24g

Notes and Variations: You can replace the bell peppers with other low FODMAP vegetables such as carrots or zucchini. If you want a bit of heat, add a sprinkle of crushed red pepper flakes.

Veggie Quesadilla

Preparation time: 15 minutes

Cooking time: 10 minutes

Servings: 2

Ingredients:

- 2 large corn tortillas (approximately 60 grams)
- 1/2 cup (about 120 grams) shredded cheddar cheese
- 1/2 cup (about 75 grams) sautéed bell peppers and zucchini

- 1 tablespoon (about 15 milliliters) garlic-infused olive oil
- A pinch of salt and pepper to taste

Directions:

1. Heat the garlic-infused olive oil in a pan over medium heat.
2. Place a tortilla in the pan, sprinkle half of the cheese on top, then spread the sautéed vegetables evenly.
3. Sprinkle the rest of the cheese on top and cover with the second tortilla.
4. Cook until the bottom tortilla is golden and crispy, then carefully flip the quesadilla and cook until the other side is golden and the cheese is melted.
5. Remove from heat and let it cool for a minute before cutting into wedges.

Nutrition: Calories: 350; Fat: 24g; Carbs: 25g; Protein: 12g

Notes and Variations: You can add cooked chicken or tofu for extra protein. Try it with a dollop of lactose-free sour cream or a splash of hot sauce for extra flavor.

Chicken and Rice Soup

Preparation time: 15 minutes

Cooking time: 45 minutes

Servings: 2

Ingredients:

- 1 boneless chicken breast (about 150 grams)
- 1 medium carrot, diced (about 60 grams)
- 1 medium zucchini, diced (about 120 grams)
- 1/2 cup of rice (about 100 grams)
- 4 cups low FODMAP chicken broth (about 950 milliliters)
- 1 tablespoon (about 15 milliliters) garlic-infused olive oil
- A pinch of salt and pepper to taste

Directions:

1. Heat the garlic-infused olive oil in a pot over medium heat.
2. Add the diced chicken breast and cook until it's no longer pink.
3. Add the diced carrot and zucchini and cook for another few minutes until the vegetables are slightly softened.
4. Add the rice and low FODMAP chicken broth. Bring to a boil.
5. Once boiling, reduce heat and simmer for about 30 minutes, until the rice is cooked and the flavors are well combined.
6. Season with salt and pepper to taste.

Nutrition: Calories: 350; Fat: 8g; Carbs: 40g; Protein: 30g

Notes and Variations: You can add other low FODMAP vegetables such as spinach or tomatoes. Try it with a squeeze of fresh lemon juice for extra flavor.

Rice Paper Rolls

| Preparation time: 20 minutes | Cooking time: 0 minutes | Servings: 2 |

Ingredients:

- 6 rice paper sheets
- 1/2 pound cooked shrimp (about 225 grams)
- 1 medium bell pepper, thinly sliced (about 120 grams)
- 1 medium carrot, peeled and thinly sliced (about 60 grams)
- 1 medium cucumber, thinly sliced (about 150 grams)

- For the peanut dipping sauce:
- 2 tablespoons peanut butter (about 32 grams)
- 1 tablespoon gluten-free soy sauce (about 15 milliliters)
- 1 tablespoon maple syrup (about 20 milliliters)

Directions:

1. Prepare the peanut dipping sauce by mixing together the peanut butter, soy sauce, and maple syrup. Set aside.
2. Dip a sheet of rice paper in warm water until it becomes soft and pliable.
3. Place a few slices of bell pepper, carrot, cucumber, and a couple of shrimp onto the middle of the rice paper.
4. Fold the sides of the rice paper in, then roll it up from the bottom, making sure the filling stays inside. Repeat with the remaining rice paper sheets and filling.
5. Serve the rice paper rolls with the peanut dipping sauce.

Nutrition: Calories: 285; Fat: 8g; Carbs: 35g; Protein: 20g

Notes and Variations: You can replace shrimp with tofu for a vegan alternative. Try it with different low FODMAP vegetables such as spinach or tomatoes.

Vegetable Omelette

| Preparation time: 10 minutes | Cooking time: 10 minutes | Servings: 1 |

Ingredients:

- 2 large eggs (about 100 grams)
- 1/4 cup diced bell pepper (about 40 grams)
- 1/4 cup diced zucchini (about 60 grams)
- 1/4 cup diced tomatoes (about 50 grams)

- 1 tablespoon olive oil (about 15 milliliters)
- A pinch of salt and pepper
- 1 tablespoon chives, chopped (about 3 grams)

Directions:

1. In a bowl, beat the eggs with a pinch of salt and pepper. Set aside.
2. Heat the olive oil in a non-stick pan over medium heat.
3. Add the bell pepper and zucchini to the pan and sauté until they start to soften.
4. Add the tomatoes to the pan and cook for another minute.
5. Pour the beaten eggs over the vegetables in the pan, tilting the pan to distribute the eggs evenly.
6. Cook the omelette until the eggs are set, then flip it over and cook for another minute.
7. Slide the omelette onto a plate and sprinkle with chopped chives.

Nutrition: Calories: 245; Fat: 19g; Carbs: 6g; Protein: 13g

Notes and Variations: You can add other low FODMAP vegetables like spinach or olives. Try it with a sprinkle of lactose-free cheese on top.

Grilled Chicken with Quinoa and Sautéed Zucchini

Preparation time: 15 minutes + chilling time

Cooking time: 20 minutes

Servings: 2

Ingredients:

- 2 boneless, skinless chicken breasts (about 500 grams)
- 2 tablespoons garlic-infused olive oil, divided (30 milliliters)
- Salt and pepper to taste

- 1 cup quinoa (185 grams)
- 2 cups water (500 milliliters)
- 2 medium zucchinis, sliced (about 400 grams)
- Lemon wedges for serving

Directions:

1. Preheat your grill to medium-high heat.
2. Rub the chicken breasts with 1 tablespoon of the garlic-infused olive oil, and season with salt and pepper.
3. Place the chicken on the grill and cook for about 6-7 minutes per side, until fully cooked through.
4. While the chicken is grilling, cook the quinoa: Rinse the quinoa under cold water, then combine it with 2 cups of water in a pot. Bring to a boil, then reduce heat to low, cover, and let simmer for about 15 minutes, until all water is absorbed.
5. In a pan, heat the remaining tablespoon of garlic-infused olive oil over medium heat. Add the zucchini slices and sauté until tender.
6. To serve, divide the cooked quinoa and zucchini among two plates, and top each with a grilled chicken breast. Serve with a lemon wedge for squeezing over the top.

Nutrition: Calories: 550; Fat: 15g; Carbs: 55g; Protein: 50g

Notes and Variations: For extra flavor, you could marinate the chicken breasts in a mixture of the garlic-infused olive oil, lemon juice, and herbs before grilling. You can substitute the zucchini with any other low FODMAP vegetables you like.

DINNER RECIPES

Baked Cod with Mashed Potatoes and Roasted Carrots

Preparation time: 15 minutes	Cooking time: 45 minutes	Servings: 1-2

Ingredients:

- 2 cod fillets (about 4-6 ounces or 113-170 grams each)
- 1 tablespoon (15 mL) olive oil
- Salt and black pepper to taste
- 2 medium-sized potatoes (about 10 ounces or 283 grams total)
- 1/4 cup (60 mL) lactose-free milk
- 2 medium-sized carrots (about 5 ounces or 141 grams total), cut into sticks
- 1 tablespoon (15 mL) olive oil for the carrots
- Salt and black pepper for the carrots

Directions:

1. Preheat your oven to 400°F (200°C) and line a baking sheet with parchment paper.
2. Place the cod fillets on the prepared baking sheet and drizzle with olive oil. Season with salt and black pepper to taste.
3. Place the cod in the oven and bake for 15-20 minutes, or until the fish flakes easily with a fork.
4. While the cod is baking, peel and dice the potatoes. Place them in a large pot, cover with water, and bring to a boil. Cook for about 15 minutes, or until the potatoes are soft.
5. Drain the potatoes and mash them with a potato masher or a fork. Add the lactose-free milk and continue mashing until you reach your desired consistency. Season with salt and black pepper to taste.
6. While the potatoes are cooking, place the carrot sticks on a baking sheet, drizzle with olive oil, and season with salt and black pepper.
7. Place in the oven and roast for about 20-25 minutes, or until the carrots are tender and slightly caramelized.
8. To serve, divide the mashed potatoes, roasted carrots, and baked cod between two plates. Serve immediately.

Nutrition: Calories: 320; Fat: 6g; Carbs: 36g; Protein: 28g

Notes and Variations: You can easily customize this recipe by using different types of fish or vegetables. For extra flavor, try adding some fresh herbs or spices to the mashed potatoes or roasted carrots.

Gluten Free Spaghetti with Marinara Sauce

Preparation time: 10 minutes	Cooking time: 20 minutes	Servings: 1-2

Ingredients:

- 4 ounces (113 grams) gluten-free spaghetti
- 1 cup (240 mL) low FODMAP marinara sauce (make sure to read the label to avoid high FODMAP ingredients)
- 2 tablespoons (30 mL) olive oil
- 1 tablespoon (15 mL) low FODMAP garlic-infused oil (for that garlic flavor without the FODMAPs)
- 1/4 cup (25 grams) freshly grated Parmesan cheese
- Salt and black pepper to taste

Directions:

1. Cook the gluten-free spaghetti according to the package instructions. When done, drain and set aside, reserving a cup of pasta water.
2. While the spaghetti is cooking, heat the olive oil and garlic-infused oil in a large pan over medium heat.
3. Add the marinara sauce to the pan and bring to a simmer. If the sauce is too thick, you can thin it out with a bit of the reserved pasta water.
4. Add the cooked and drained spaghetti to the pan and toss until it's fully coated in the sauce. Season with salt and black pepper to taste.
5. To serve, divide the spaghetti between two plates and sprinkle with the freshly grated Parmesan cheese. Serve immediately.

Nutrition: Calories: 350; Fat: 12g; Carbs: 50g; Protein: 10g

Notes and Variations: Make sure to use a gluten-free spaghetti that you enjoy, as not all gluten-free pastas are created equal.. If you're not a fan of Parmesan, you could also top your spaghetti with a bit of lactose-free ricotta or mozzarella cheese.

Veggie Pizza on a Gluten Free Crust

Preparation time: 15 minutes

Cooking time: 15-20 minutes

Servings: 1-2

Ingredients:

- 1 small gluten-free pizza base (about 9 inches or 23 cm in diameter)
- 1/4 cup (60 mL) low FODMAP tomato sauce
- 1/2 bell pepper (red or green), thinly sliced
- 2 tablespoons (30 mL) sliced black olives
- 1/2 cup (50 grams) shredded mozzarella cheese
- Olive oil, for drizzling
- Salt and black pepper, to taste
- Fresh basil leaves, for garnish (optional)

Directions:

1. Preheat your oven according to the instructions on the gluten-free pizza base packaging.
2. Place the pizza base on a baking sheet or pizza stone.

3. Spread the tomato sauce evenly over the pizza base, leaving a small border for the crust.
4. Arrange the thinly sliced bell pepper and black olives over the sauce.
5. Sprinkle the shredded mozzarella cheese evenly over the top.
6. Drizzle a little olive oil over the pizza and season with salt and black pepper.
7. Bake in the preheated oven according to the pizza base instructions, usually for around 15-20 minutes, or until the cheese is bubbly and golden.
8. Remove from the oven and allow to cool slightly before slicing. Garnish with fresh basil leaves if desired. Serve immediately.

Nutrition: Calories: 300; Fat: 10g; Carbs: 45g; Protein: 10g

Notes and Variations: You can add other low FODMAP veggies such as spinach or cherry tomatoes for added flavor and nutrition. For a lactose-free version, use lactose-free mozzarella or another lactose-free cheese of your choice.

Lemon and Thyme Roasted Turkey Breast

Preparation time: 15 minutes

Cooking time: 45-55 minutes

Servings: 1-2

Ingredients:

- 1 turkey breast (about 1 lb or 450 grams)
- 1 lemon, zested and juiced (approximately 2 tablespoons (30 mL) juice and 1 tablespoon (15 mL) zest)
- 2 tablespoons (30 mL) olive oil
- 1 teaspoon (5 mL) dried thyme
- Salt and black pepper, to taste
- Fresh thyme sprigs, for garnish (optional)

Directions:

1. Preheat your oven to 375°F (190°C).
2. Place the turkey breast in a roasting pan.
3. In a small bowl, mix together the lemon zest, lemon juice, olive oil, dried thyme, salt, and pepper.
4. Rub the lemon-thyme mixture all over the turkey breast.
5. Roast in the preheated oven for about 45-55 minutes, or until the turkey is cooked through and the juices run clear. The internal temperature should reach 165°F (74°C) on a meat thermometer.
6. Remove from the oven and let rest for 10 minutes before slicing.

Nutrition: Calories: 300; Fat: 7g; Carbs: 2g; Protein: 56g

Notes and Variations: For a more robust flavor, consider adding minced garlic to the lemon-thyme mixture. Garlic-infused olive oil is a great option as well, as it provides flavor without the high FODMAPs.

Spaghetti Bolognese with Gluten-Free Pasta

Preparation time: 15 minutes

Cooking time: 45 minutes

Servings: 1-2

Ingredients:

- 2 cups (approx. 120g) gluten-free spaghetti
- 1/2 lb (approx. 225g) ground beef or turkey
- 1 medium carrot, finely chopped (approx. 64g)
- 1 stick of celery, finely chopped (approx. 64g)
- 2 tablespoons (approx. 30 mL) olive oil
- 1/2 cup (approx. 125 mL) canned tomatoes
- Salt and black pepper, to taste
- 2 tablespoons (approx. 30 mL) low FODMAP beef broth
- 1 tablespoon (approx. 15 mL) garlic-infused olive oil
- 1/2 cup (approx. 50g) grated Parmesan cheese, for serving

Directions:

1. Heat the olive oil in a large skillet over medium heat. Add the ground beef and cook until browned. Remove from the skillet and set aside.
2. In the same skillet, add the finely chopped carrot and celery. Cook until soft.
3. Return the ground beef to the skillet. Add the canned tomatoes and beef broth. Season with salt and pepper.
4. Lower the heat and simmer the sauce for about 30 minutes, or until it has thickened.
5. While the sauce is simmering, cook the gluten-free spaghetti according to the package instructions. Drain well.
6. Drizzle the garlic-infused olive oil over the drained pasta and toss to coat.
7. Serve the spaghetti topped with the Bolognese sauce. Sprinkle with grated Parmesan cheese before serving.

Nutrition: Calories: 600; Fat: 25g; Carbs: 60g; Protein: 30g

Notes and Variations: You can add a touch of red wine to the Bolognese sauce for extra flavor. Ensure you simmer the sauce well to allow the alcohol to cook off. Feel free to add other low FODMAP vegetables to the Bolognese sauce, such as bell peppers or zucchini. Remember to choose a gluten-free pasta that is made with low FODMAP ingredients. Some gluten-free pastas may contain high FODMAP ingredients like lentils or soy.

Lambs Chops with Rosemary and Garlic Infused Oil

Preparation time: 15 minutes

Cooking time: 15 minutes

Servings: 1-2

Ingredients:

- 2 lamb chops (approx. 250g)
- 1 tablespoon fresh rosemary, finely chopped (approx. 3g)
- 2 tablespoons garlic-infused olive oil (approx. 30 mL)
- Salt and black pepper, to taste
- 1 tablespoon lemon juice (approx. 15 mL)

Directions:

1. Preheat a grill or skillet over medium-high heat.
2. Rub the lamb chops with the garlic-infused olive oil, then season them with the chopped rosemary, salt, and pepper.
3. Place the lamb chops on the grill or in the skillet. Cook for about 4-5 minutes on each side, or until they reach your desired level of doneness.
4. Once cooked, remove the lamb chops from the heat and let them rest for a few minutes.
5. Drizzle with lemon juice before serving.

Nutrition: Calories: 485; Fat: 32g; Carbs: 1g; Protein: 45g

Notes and Variations: Pair these lamb chops with a side of roasted low FODMAP vegetables or a simple green salad. For more intense flavor, consider marinating the lamb chops in the garlic-infused oil and rosemary for a few hours before cooking.

Ratatouille with Eggplant, Zucchini, and Tomatoes

Preparation time: 20 minutes

Cooking time: 60 minutes

Servings: 1-2

Ingredients:

- 1 medium eggplant (approx. 500g), cut into cubes
- 1 medium zucchini (approx. 200g), cut into cubes
- 1 cup canned tomatoes (approx. 240g)
- 1 tablespoon garlic-infused olive oil (approx. 15mL)
- 1 teaspoon fresh thyme leaves (approx. 1g)
- Salt and black pepper, to taste

Directions:

1. Preheat your oven to 375°F (190°C).
2. In a large bowl, toss the eggplant and zucchini cubes with the garlic-infused olive oil, thyme, salt, and pepper.
3. Spread the vegetables out in a single layer on a baking sheet.
4. Roast for about 30 minutes, then add the canned tomatoes and mix well.
5. Continue roasting for another 30 minutes, or until the vegetables are tender and lightly browned.

6. Once cooked, remove from the oven and adjust the seasoning if necessary before serving.

Nutrition: Calories: 140; Fat: 3g; Carbs: 27g; Protein: 5g

Notes and Variations: Ratatouille is traditionally served as a side dish, but you can also serve it as a main dish over rice or quinoa for a satisfying vegetarian meal. You can add other low FODMAP vegetables like bell peppers or olives to this dish, if you'd like.

Grilled Tuna Steak with a Sesame and Ginger Marinade

Preparation time: 10 minutes+ 30 minutes marinating time

Cooking time: 8 minutes

Servings: 1-2

Ingredients:

- 2 small tuna steaks (approx. 150g each or 5.3 oz each)
- 2 tablespoons sesame oil (approx. 30mL)
- 1 tablespoon fresh ginger, grated (approx. 6g)
- 2 tablespoons gluten-free soy sauce (approx. 30mL)
- 1 tablespoon lime juice (approx. 15mL)
- 1 tablespoon green onion tops (green parts only), finely chopped (approx. 6g)
- - Sesame seeds, for garnish

Directions:

1. In a bowl, mix together the sesame oil, grated ginger, soy sauce, and lime juice.
2. Place the tuna steaks in the marinade, making sure they're fully covered. Leave to marinate in the refrigerator for at least 30 minutes.
3. Preheat your grill to high heat.
4. Remove the tuna steaks from the marinade, pat dry, and grill each side for approximately 3-4 minutes for medium-rare, or until cooked to your preference.
5. Garnish with the chopped green onion tops and sesame seeds before serving.

Nutrition: Calories: 370; Fat: 20g; Carbs: 3g; Protein: 40g

Notes and Variations: You can replace the tuna with salmon or chicken, but cooking times will vary. If you're not a fan of raw green onions, you can lightly sauté them in a pan with a bit of oil until they're soft. For added vegetables, serve this with a side of stir-fried bell peppers or zucchini.

Beef Stew with Carrots and Parsnips

Preparation time: 15 minutes

Cooking time: 2 hours

Servings: 1-2

Ingredients:

- 200g (or 7 ounces) stewing beef, cut into bite-sized pieces
- 1 tablespoon vegetable oil (approx. 15mL)
- 2 medium carrots (approx. 120g or 4.2 ounces), cut into chunks
- 2 medium parsnips (approx. 170g or 6 ounces), cut into chunks
- 2 cups beef broth, low-sodium and gluten-free (approx. 470mL)
- 1 bay leaf
- Salt and pepper, to taste
- Fresh parsley, chopped (for garnish)

Directions:

1. Heat the oil in a large pot over medium-high heat.
2. Season the beef with salt and pepper, then add to the pot. Cook until all sides are browned, about 5-7 minutes. Remove the beef and set aside.
3. In the same pot, add the carrots and parsnips, cook for about 5 minutes until they start to soften.
4. Return the beef to the pot, add the beef broth and bay leaf. Bring to a simmer.
5. Reduce the heat to low, cover, and let it cook for about 2 hours, or until the beef is tender.
6. Check the seasoning and adjust if necessary. Remove the bay leaf.
7. Serve the stew hot, garnished with chopped parsley.

Nutrition: Calories: 470; Fat: 23g; Carbs: 28g; Protein: 35g

Notes and Variations: You can add other low FODMAP vegetables like zucchini or spinach towards the end of the cooking time. You can serve this stew with a side of mashed potatoes or a slice of gluten-free bread.

Baked Trout with Lemon, served with Quinoa

Preparation time: 10 minutes   Cooking time: 20 minutes   Servings: 1-2

Ingredients:

- 1 trout fillet (approx. 150g or 5.3 ounces)
- 1 lemon (approx. 100g or 3.5 ounces), sliced
- 2 tablespoons of olive oil (approx. 30mL)
- Salt and pepper, to taste
- 1 cup quinoa (approx. 185g or 6.5 ounces)
- 2 cups water (approx. 470mL)

Directions:

1. Preheat your oven to 200°C (or 392°F).

2. Rinse the quinoa under cold water until the water runs clear. In a saucepan, bring the water to a boil, add the quinoa, reduce the heat to low, cover, and let it simmer for about 15 minutes, or until the quinoa is cooked and fluffy. Set aside.
3. While the quinoa is cooking, season the trout fillet with salt, pepper, and 1 tablespoon of olive oil. Place the fillet on a baking sheet lined with parchment paper, arrange the lemon slices on top.
4. Bake the trout in the preheated oven for about 10-15 minutes, or until the fish is cooked through and flakes easily with a fork.
5. Serve the trout hot, drizzled with the remaining olive oil, and a side of the cooked quinoa.

Nutrition: Calories: 210; Fat: 12g; Carbs: 16g; Protein: 10g

Notes and Variations: You can add some fresh herbs like dill or parsley to the trout before baking for extra flavor.If you prefer, you can replace the quinoa with a side of steamed vegetables or a green salad.

Roasted Chicken with Thyme, served with Mashed Potatoes

Preparation time: 15minutes

Cooking time: 1 hour 15 minutes

Servings: 1-2

Ingredients:

- 2 chicken breasts (about 300g or 10.6 ounces)
- 1 tablespoon fresh thyme leaves (or 1 teaspoon dried thyme)
- 2 tablespoons of olive oil (approx. 30mL)
- Salt and pepper, to taste

- 2 medium russet potatoes (approx. 300g or 10.6 ounces)
- 2 tablespoons lactose-free butter (approx. 30g)
- 1/4 cup lactose-free milk (approx. 60mL)

Directions:

1. Preheat your oven to 200°C (or 392°F).
2. Season the chicken breasts with salt, pepper, thyme, and 1 tablespoon of olive oil. Place the chicken breasts on a baking sheet lined with parchment paper.
3. Bake the chicken in the preheated oven for about 25-30 minutes, or until the chicken is cooked through and no longer pink in the center.
4. While the chicken is cooking, peel the potatoes and cut them into equal-sized chunks. Place the potatoes in a saucepan, cover with water, add a pinch of salt, and bring to a boil. Reduce the heat to low and let the potatoes simmer until they are soft and easily pierced with a fork, about 15-20 minutes.
5. Drain the potatoes and return them to the saucepan. Add the lactose-free butter and milk, and mash until smooth. Season with salt and pepper to taste.
6. Serve the roasted chicken hot, drizzled with the remaining olive oil, and a side of the mashed potatoes.

Nutrition: Calories: 620; Fat: 20g; Carbs: 50g; Protein: 50g

Notes and Variations: You can add other herbs and spices to the chicken before roasting, such as rosemary, garlic-infused oil, or paprika.

Gluten-Free Pasta with Olive Oil, Chili Flakes, and Parmesan Cheese

Preparation time: 5 minutes

Cooking time: 15 minutes

Servings: 1-2

Ingredients:

- 2 servings gluten-free pasta (about 200g or 7 ounces)
- 3 tablespoons olive oil (approx. 45mL)
- 1/2 teaspoon red chili flakes
- 1/4 cup Parmesan cheese, grated (approx. 25g)
- Salt, to taste

Directions:
1. Cook the gluten-free pasta according to the package instructions in a pot of boiling, salted water. Drain the pasta, reserving a little bit of the pasta water for later use.
2. In a large pan, heat the olive oil over medium heat. Add the red chili flakes to the oil, stirring to distribute the heat of the flakes through the oil.
3. Add the cooked pasta to the pan, tossing it in the chili-infused oil to ensure it is fully coated.
4. If the pasta seems a bit dry, add some of the reserved pasta water.
5. Take the pan off the heat, add the grated Parmesan cheese, and toss the pasta again until it's well mixed and the cheese has melted into the pasta.
6. Season with additional salt if needed, then serve immediately.

Nutrition: Calories: 635; Fat: 25g; Carbs: 85g; Protein: 15g

Notes and Variations: Always check the label of your gluten-free pasta to ensure no high FODMAP ingredients are present.

Lemon and Herb Roasted Chicken with Steamed Carrots

Preparation time: 15 minutes

Cooking time: 90 minutes

Servings: 2

Ingredients:

- 1 small whole chicken (about 2 to 3 pounds, or 1 to 1.3 kilograms)
- 2 tablespoons olive oil (30 mL)
- - Juice of 1 lemon
- 1 tablespoon garlic-infused oil

- 1 teaspoon dried thyme
- 1 teaspoon dried rosemary
- Salt and pepper to taste

- 2 medium carrots (about 1 cup when cut, or 128 grams), cut into batons
- 1 tablespoon unsalted butter (15 grams)

Directions:

1. Preheat your oven to 375°F (190°C).
2. In a small bowl, mix together the olive oil, lemon juice, garlic-infused oil, thyme, rosemary, salt, and pepper.
3. Rinse the chicken and pat it dry. Brush the chicken all over with the herb and oil mixture.
4. Place the chicken in a roasting pan and cook in the preheated oven for approximately 1.5 hours, or until the internal temperature reaches 165°F (74°C).
5. While the chicken is roasting, steam the carrots until they are tender. This should take about 15-20 minutes.
6. Toss the steamed carrots with the butter, and season with salt and pepper.

Nutrition: Calories: 415; Fat: 27g; Carbs: 8g; Protein: 35g

Notes and Variations: The roasting time for the chicken may vary depending on its size. Always ensure the chicken is fully cooked to avoid foodborne illness. You can replace the carrots with other low FODMAP vegetables such as zucchini or bell peppers.

Grilled Tuna Steak
with a Soy and Ginger Marinade

Preparation time: 10 minutes

Cooking time: 10 minutes

Servings: 2

Ingredients:

- 2 tuna steaks (about 6 oz each, or 170 grams each)
- 2 tablespoons of garlic-infused oil (30 mL)
- 1 tablespoon of fresh ginger, finely grated (about 6 grams)

- 2 tablespoons of gluten-free soy sauce (30 mL)
- 1 tablespoon of fresh lemon juice (15 mL)
- Salt and pepper to taste

Directions:

1. In a bowl, mix the garlic-infused oil, grated ginger, soy sauce, and lemon juice to create the marinade.
2. Season the tuna steaks with salt and pepper, then place them in a dish. Pour the marinade over the tuna steaks and turn them to coat evenly. Allow them to marinate in the refrigerator for at least 30 minutes.
3. Preheat your grill or grill pan over medium-high heat.

4. Grill the tuna steaks for 4-5 minutes per side, until they're cooked to your desired level of doneness.
5. Serve the tuna steaks with a side of steamed vegetables or a green salad.

Nutrition: Calories: 220; Fat: 5g; Carbs: 2g; Protein: 40g

Notes and Variations: You can substitute the soy sauce for a gluten-free tamari if you prefer.If you don't have fresh ginger, you can use 1/2 teaspoon of dried ginger powder.

Turkey Tacos

Preparation time: 15 minutes	Cooking time: 20 minutes	Servings: 2

Ingredients:

- 8 ounces ground turkey (around 225 grams)
- 4 corn tortillas
- 1 tablespoon garlic-infused oil (15 mL)
- 1/2 teaspoon ground cumin (2.5 mL)
- 1/2 teaspoon ground coriander (2.5 mL)
- 1/4 teaspoon smoked paprika (1.25 mL)
- Salt and pepper to taste
- 1 cup chopped lettuce (50 grams)
- 1 medium tomato, diced (about 123 grams)

Directions:

1. Heat the garlic-infused oil in a large pan over medium heat. Add the ground turkey, breaking it up with a spoon as it cooks. Cook until it's no longer pink, about 7-10 minutes.
2. Stir in the cumin, coriander, paprika, salt, and pepper, cooking for another minute until the turkey is well-coated in the spices.
3. Warm up the corn tortillas in a dry pan over medium heat, or in the microwave covered with a damp paper towel.
4. To assemble the tacos, divide the cooked ground turkey evenly between the tortillas. Top with the chopped lettuce and diced tomato.
5. Serve immediately, with a side of low FODMAP salsa if desired.

Nutrition: Calories: 330; Fat: 12g; Carbs: 22g; Protein: 28g

Notes and Variations: For a vegetarian version, substitute the ground turkey with a low FODMAP serving of canned lentils or chickpeas.

Beef and Vegetable Skewers

Preparation time: 15 minutes	Cooking time: 15 minutes + marination time (2 hours)	Servings: 2

Ingredients:

- 8 ounces of lean beef, cut into 1-inch cubes (about 225 grams)
- 1 medium zucchini, cut into 1-inch chunks
- 1 red bell pepper, cut into 1-inch squares
- 1 tablespoon garlic-infused oil (15 mL)
- 1 tablespoon lemon juice (15 mL)
- 1 teaspoon dried oregano (5 mL)
- Salt and pepper to taste
- 4 wooden skewers, soaked in water for 30 minutes before use

Directions:

1. In a bowl, combine the garlic-infused oil, lemon juice, dried oregano, salt, and pepper to make the marinade.
2. Add the beef cubes to the marinade, mix well to coat. Cover and refrigerate for at least 2 hours.
3. Preheat your grill to medium-high heat.
4. Thread the marinated beef, bell pepper, and zucchini onto the skewers, alternating between each ingredient.
5. Grill the skewers for 12-15 minutes, turning occasionally until the beef is cooked to your liking and the vegetables are tender.
6. Remove from the grill and let rest for a few minutes before serving.

Nutrition: Calories: 310; Fat: 16g; Carbs: 7g; Protein: 34g

Notes and Variations: Be careful when using garlic-infused oil, as some products may contain actual garlic pieces, which are high in FODMAPs. Always choose an oil that has been made with the infusion method and doesn't contain any floating pieces of garlic.

Maple Glazed Salmon with Quinoa and Steamed Vegetables

Preparation time: 15 minutes

Cooking time: 20 minutes

Servings: 1-2

Ingredients:

- 1 salmon filet (approximately 6 oz or 170 grams)
- 2 tablespoons pure maple syrup (30 ml)
- 1 cup quinoa (170 grams)
- 2 cups of water (480 ml)
- Assorted vegetables for steaming (such as zucchini, carrots, and bell peppers)
- Salt and pepper to taste
- 1 tablespoon of olive oil (15 ml)

Directions:

1. Rinse the quinoa under cold water until the water runs clear. Place it in a pot with the water and bring it to a boil. Once boiling, reduce the heat to low, cover the pot, and let it simmer for about 15 minutes until the quinoa is cooked.

2. Preheat your oven to 400°F (200°C). Place the salmon on a baking sheet lined with foil.
3. In a small bowl, combine the maple syrup, salt, and pepper. Brush the glaze over the salmon filet.
4. Bake the salmon for about 15-20 minutes, or until it flakes easily with a fork.
5. While the salmon is baking, chop your vegetables and steam them until they are tender, about 10-15 minutes.
6. Once everything is cooked, serve the salmon over a bed of quinoa, with the steamed vegetables on the side. Drizzle with olive oil and season with additional salt and pepper if desired.

Nutrition: Calories: 530; Fat: 15g; Carbs: 60g; Protein: 42g

Notes and Variations: You can replace the salmon with another type of fish like trout or tilapia. Feel free to mix and match the vegetables based on what you have available. Remember to check that your maple syrup is pure and doesn't contain any high FODMAP ingredients like high-fructose corn syrup. You can also grill the salmon instead of baking it for a different flavor profile.

Low FODMAP Chicken Tacos

Preparation time: 15 minutes

Cooking time: 15 minutes

Servings: 1-2

Ingredients:

- 1 medium chicken breast, grilled and sliced (around 170 grams)
- 2 small lettuce leaves, shredded (approx. 15 grams)
- 2 medium tomatoes, diced (approx. 123 grams)
- 1/4 cup of cheddar cheese, grated (approx. 28 grams)
- 2 corn tortillas (approx. 50 grams)

Directions:

1. Preheat your grill or grill pan over medium heat. Season the chicken breast with salt and pepper, then grill for about 6-7 minutes per side, or until fully cooked. Remove from the grill and let it rest for a few minutes, then slice into strips.
2. Warm the corn tortillas in a dry skillet over medium heat, or directly over the flame of a gas stove, until they're soft and pliable.
3. To assemble the tacos, spread the shredded lettuce on each tortilla, then top with the grilled chicken strips, diced tomatoes, and a sprinkle of cheddar cheese.

Nutrition: Calories: 460; Fat: 14g; Carbs: 33g; Protein: 50g

Notes and Variations: You can add a drizzle of low FODMAP salsa or a squeeze of lime for extra flavor. For a vegetarian version, replace the chicken with grilled tofu or a low FODMAP bean, such as chickpeas.

Low FODMAP Vegetable Frittata

Preparation time: 10 minutes + resting time

Cooking time: 20 minutes

Servings: 2

Ingredients:

- 4 large eggs
- 1/2 bell pepper, chopped (about 75g)
- 1/2 zucchini, chopped (about 120g)
- 50g feta cheese, crumbled
- A small handful of fresh herbs (such as parsley or chives), finely chopped
- Salt and pepper, to taste
- 1 tablespoon olive oil

Directions:

1. Preheat the oven to 180°C (356°F).
2. In a medium-sized bowl, beat the eggs and mix in the feta cheese, fresh herbs, salt, and pepper. Set aside.
3. Heat the olive oil in an ovenproof skillet over medium heat.
4. Add the bell pepper and zucchini to the skillet and cook for about 5 minutes, until they begin to soften.
5. Pour the egg mixture over the vegetables in the skillet, ensuring an even distribution. Let it cook on the stovetop for about 2-3 minutes without stirring, until the edges start to set.
6. Transfer the skillet to the preheated oven and bake for about 10-15 minutes, until the frittata is set and golden brown.
7. Allow it to cool slightly, then slice and serve with a side salad.

Nutrition: Calories: 220; Fat: 16g; Carbs: 6g; Protein: 15g

Notes and Variations: You can mix and match your favorite low-FODMAP vegetables in this recipe. Some good options include spinach, olives, or cherry tomatoes. For a dairy-free version, omit the feta cheese or replace it with a lactose-free cheese of your choice.

Sesame Ginger Shrimp Stir-fry

Preparation time: 15 minutes

Cooking time: 10 minutes

Servings: 2

Ingredients:

- 300g shrimp, peeled and deveined (about 10 ounces)
- 1/2 bell pepper, sliced (about 75g)
- 1 carrot, sliced (about 60g)
- 1/2 zucchini, sliced (about 120g)
- 2 tablespoons gluten-free soy sauce (30 ml)
- 1 tablespoon fresh ginger, finely chopped (about 15g)

- 1 tablespoon sesame seeds (about 9g)
- 2 tablespoons sesame oil (30 ml)

Directions:

1. In a small bowl, combine the soy sauce and finely chopped ginger. Set aside.
2. Heat 1 tablespoon of sesame oil in a large frying pan over medium-high heat.
3. Add the shrimp to the pan and sauté for about 2-3 minutes on each side, until they are pink and cooked through. Remove the shrimp from the pan and set aside.
4. In the same pan, add another tablespoon of sesame oil. Add the bell pepper, carrot, and zucchini to the pan, stirring frequently. Cook for about 5-7 minutes, until the vegetables are tender.
5. Return the shrimp to the pan with the vegetables. Pour the soy sauce and ginger mixture over the top, stirring to combine. Cook for another 2 minutes until everything is heated through.
6. Sprinkle with sesame seeds just before serving.

Nutrition: Calories: 350; Fat: 22g; Carbs: 10g; Protein: 24

Gluten-Free Pasta with Olive Oil and Garlic

Preparation time: 10 minutes   Cooking time: 20 minutes   Servings: 1-2

Ingredients:

- 1 cup of gluten-free pasta (about 100 grams)
- 2 tablespoons of garlic-infused olive oil (30 ml)
- 1/4 cup chopped fresh parsley (about 15 grams)
- 2 tablespoons of freshly grated Parmesan cheese (10 grams)
- Salt and black pepper to taste

Directions:

1. Bring a large pot of salted water to a boil. Add the gluten-free pasta and cook according to the package instructions until al dente.
2. While the pasta is cooking, heat the garlic-infused olive oil in a large skillet over medium heat.
3. Drain the pasta, reserving a little bit of the pasta water.
4. Add the drained pasta to the skillet with the garlic-infused olive oil. Toss to coat the pasta in the oil. If the pasta seems a little dry, add a bit of the reserved pasta water.
5. Season the pasta with salt and black pepper to taste.
6. Stir in the chopped fresh parsley and the freshly grated Parmesan cheese. Toss until the pasta is well coated in the cheese and parsley.
7. Serve immediately. Enjoy your low FODMAP meal!

Nutrition: Calories: 500; Fat: 20g; Carbs: 70g; Protein: 15g

Notes and Variations: This recipe is also great with added cooked chicken or shrimp for a protein boost. You can add some chili flakes for a spicy kick.

Grilled Shrimp Skewers

Preparation time: 15 minutes + 30 for marinating

Cooking time: 10 minutes

Servings: 1-2

Ingredients:

- 12 large shrimp, peeled and deveined (about 200 grams)
- 2 tablespoons of garlic-infused olive oil (30 ml)
- Juice and zest of 1 lemon
- Salt and black pepper to taste
- 4 skewers

Directions:

1. In a bowl, mix together the garlic-infused olive oil, lemon juice, and lemon zest. Add the shrimp and toss to coat. Let the shrimp marinate in the refrigerator for at least 30 minutes.
2. Preheat your grill to medium-high heat.
3. Thread the shrimp onto the skewers. Season with salt and black pepper.
4. Grill the shrimp skewers for 2-3 minutes on each side, until the shrimp are pink and cooked through.
5. Serve immediately, with a wedge of lemon if desired. Enjoy your low FODMAP meal!

Nutrition: Calories: 250; Fat: 7g; Carbs: 2g; Protein: 46g

Notes and Variations: Always ensure your shrimp is fresh and properly cleaned before using. You can add some chopped fresh herbs like parsley or dill to the marinade for additional flavor. These skewers can be served with a side of low FODMAP salad or grilled vegetables for a complete meal. You can also use this marinade with other types of seafood like scallops or fish.

Beef and Vegetable Kebabs

Preparation time: 20 minutes

Cooking time: 15 minutes

Servings: 2

Ingredients:

- 1/2 pound of beef cubes (around 227 grams)
- 1 medium bell pepper
- 1 medium zucchini
- 2 tablespoons of garlic-infused olive oil (30 ml)
- 1 tablespoon of tamari or gluten-free soy sauce (15 ml)
- 1 teaspoon of paprika
- Salt and black pepper to taste
- 4 skewers

Directions:

1. In a bowl, mix together the garlic-infused olive oil, tamari or gluten-free soy sauce, paprika, salt, and black pepper. Add the beef cubes and toss to coat. Cover and marinate in the refrigerator for at least 2 hours.
2. Preheat your grill to medium-high heat.
3. Cut the bell pepper and zucchini into chunks.
4. Thread the marinated beef cubes and vegetable chunks onto the skewers, alternating between the beef and vegetables.
1. Grill the kebabs for about 10-15 minutes, turning occasionally, until the beef is cooked to your liking and the vegetables are tender.
2. Serve immediately.

Nutrition: Calories: 430; Fat: 32g; Carbs: 9g; Protein: 26g

Notes and Variations: Ensure the beef is cooked thoroughly to prevent foodborne illnesses. You can also use other low FODMAP vegetables like tomatoes or eggplants. For a complete meal, serve these kebabs with a side of low FODMAP rice or quinoa.

Tomato and Basil Frittata

Preparation time: 10 minutes

Cooking time: 15 minutes

Servings: 2

Ingredients:

- 4 large eggs
- 1 medium tomato (around 123 grams)
- 1/4 cup fresh basil leaves (about 15 grams)
- 1 tablespoon of garlic-infused olive oil (15 ml)
- Salt and black pepper to taste

Directions:

1. Preheat the oven to 350°F (180°C).
2. Crack the eggs into a bowl, season with salt and pepper, and beat well.
3. Chop the tomato and tear the basil leaves into small pieces.
4. Heat the garlic-infused olive oil in an ovenproof skillet over medium heat.
5. Add the chopped tomato to the skillet and cook for a few minutes until softened.
6. Pour the beaten eggs over the tomato in the skillet, then sprinkle the torn basil leaves on top.
7. Cook the frittata for a few minutes until the edges start to set, then transfer the skillet to the preheated oven.
8. Bake for 10-15 minutes until the frittata is fully set.
9. Remove from the oven, let it cool for a few minutes, then cut into wedges and serve.

Nutrition: Calories: 210; Fat: 15g; Carbs: 4g; Protein: 13g

Notes and Variations: For a cheesy variation, sprinkle a small amount of a low FODMAP cheese, like feta or mozzarella, on top of the frittata before baking.

Ginger and Scallion Chicken Stir-Fry

Preparation time: 10 minutes

Cooking time: 20 minutes

Servings: 2

Ingredients:

- 1 large chicken breast (about 200 grams)
- 1 inch piece of fresh ginger (about 25 grams)
- 2 scallions, green part only (about 30 grams)
- 1 bell pepper (about 120 grams)
- 1 zucchini (about 200 grams)
- 2 tablespoons of low-sodium soy sauce (30 ml)
- 1 tablespoon of garlic-infused olive oil (15 ml)
- Salt and black pepper to taste

Directions:

1. Slice the chicken breast into thin strips.
2. Peel and slice the ginger. Slice the scallion greens and the bell pepper. Cut the zucchini into half-moons.
3. Heat the garlic-infused olive oil in a large frying pan or wok over medium heat.
4. Add the chicken strips to the pan and stir-fry for a few minutes until they are no longer pink in the middle.
5. Add the sliced ginger, scallion greens, bell pepper, and zucchini to the pan.
6. Stir-fry the vegetables and chicken for a few more minutes until the vegetables are tender-crisp.
7. Add the low-sodium soy sauce to the pan, season with salt and pepper, and toss everything together until well mixed.
8. Cook for a minute or two more, then serve the stir-fry hot.

Nutrition: Calories: 330; Fat: 16g; Carbs: 10g; Protein: 35g

Notes and Variations: For more heat, add a sliced red chili or a sprinkle of crushed red pepper flakes to the stir-fry.

Baked Cod with Green Beans

Preparation time: 10 minutes

Cooking time: 15 minutes

Servings: 2

Ingredients:

- 2 cod fillets (about 6 ounces or 170 grams each)
- 2 cups green beans (about 200 grams)
- 2 lemons

- 2 tablespoons olive oil (30 ml)
- Salt and pepper to taste

Directions:

1. Preheat the oven to 400°F (200°C).
2. Rinse the green beans and trim the ends. Rinse the cod fillets and pat dry with a paper towel.
3. Arrange the green beans and cod fillets on a baking sheet. Drizzle with olive oil and squeeze the juice of one lemon over top. Season with salt and pepper.
4. Thinly slice the remaining lemon and arrange the slices on top of the cod fillets.
5. Bake for 12-15 minutes, or until the cod is opaque and flaky and the green beans are tender.
6. Serve hot, with additional lemon wedges if desired.

Nutrition: Calories: 250; Fat: 8g; Carbs: 12g; Protein: 35g

Notes and Variations: You can also add other low FODMAP vegetables to the baking sheet, such as bell peppers or zucchini. If you want to add more flavor, you can sprinkle some dried herbs like dill or parsley over the cod before baking.

Poached Cod with Parsley Sauce

Preparation time: 10 minutes

Cooking time: 15 minutes

Servings: 2

Ingredients:

- 2 cod fillets (about 6 ounces or 170 grams each)
- 2 cups of water (475 ml)
- 1 cup fresh parsley leaves (about 60 grams)
- 1/4 cup garlic-infused olive oil (60 ml)
- Salt and pepper to taste

Directions:

1. In a large skillet, bring the water to a simmer. Add the cod fillets and cook gently for 7-10 minutes, or until the fish is opaque and flaky.
2. While the fish is cooking, make the parsley sauce. In a blender or food processor, combine the parsley leaves, garlic-infused olive oil, salt, and pepper. Blend until smooth.
3. Remove the fish from the skillet and drain on a paper towel.
4. To serve, plate the fish and drizzle the parsley sauce over top.

Nutrition: Calories: 300; Fat: 15g; Carbs: 1g; Protein: 35g

Notes and Variations: You can serve this dish with a side of boiled potatoes or a simple salad for a complete meal. Feel free to use other herbs like dill or cilantro instead of parsley. To add some heat, add a pinch of chili flakes to the parsley sauce.

Grilled Steak with Baked Potatoes

Preparation time: 10 minutes

Cooking time: 20 minutes

Servings: 2

Ingredients:

- 2 steak cuts (around 8 ounces or 225 grams each)
- 2 medium russet potatoes (about 5 ounces or 140 grams each)
- 2 tablespoons of olive oil (30 ml)
- Salt and pepper to taste

Directions:

1. Preheat your grill and oven to medium-high heat.
2. Rub the steaks with a tablespoon of olive oil, and season with salt and pepper to taste.
3. Pierce the potatoes with a fork a few times to create small holes, then rub them with the remaining olive oil.
4. Place the potatoes in the oven and bake for about 45-60 minutes, or until they're soft and cooked through.
5. While the potatoes are baking, grill the steaks to your desired level of doneness. This will typically take about 4-5 minutes per side for medium-rare.
6. Let the steaks rest for a few minutes before serving.
7. Serve each steak with a baked potato on the side.

Nutrition: Calories: 600; Fat: 20g; Carbs: 4g; Protein: 50g

Notes and Variations: For additional flavor, you can add garlic or rosemary to your steaks while they're grilling. To check the doneness of your steak, use a meat thermometer: 120-130°F (49-54°C) for rare, 135-140°F (57-60°C) for medium-rare, 145-150°F (63-66°C) for medium, and 155-160°F (68-71°C) for well-done. The baking time for the potatoes can vary depending on their size, so check them for doneness by inserting a fork into the center. If it goes in easily, the potato is done.

SWEET DESSERTS

Strawberry Sorbet

Preparation time: 15 minutes

Freezing Time: 4 hours or overnight

Servings: 2

Ingredients:

2 cups strawberries, hulled (about 300g)

- 1/2 cup granulated sugar (about 100g)

- - 1 tablespoon lemon juice (about 15ml
-

Directions:

1. Rinse, hull, and quarter the strawberries.
2. In a blender, combine the strawberries, sugar, and lemon juice. Blend until smooth.
3. Pour the mixture through a fine-mesh strainer into a bowl to remove the seeds. Discard the seeds.
4. Transfer the strained mixture into a shallow dish suitable for freezing.
5. Freeze the mixture for 4 hours or overnight, until it is completely solid.
6. Before serving, let the sorbet sit at room temperature for a few minutes to soften slightly. Use a spoon or an ice cream scoop to serve.

Nutrition: Calories: 236; Fat: 0g; Carbs: 60g; Protein: 1g

Notes and Variations: The sugar can be replaced with a suitable low FODMAP sweetener if desired, but this may affect the texture and freezing point of the sorbet. You can also try this recipe with other low FODMAP fruits like blueberries or raspberries.

Almond Milk Rice Pudding

Preparation time: 10 minutes

Cooking time: 40 minutes

Servings: 2

Ingredients:

- 1/2 cup short grain white rice (about 100g)
- 2 cups almond milk (about 500ml)
- 1/4 cup granulated sugar (about 50g)
- 1/2 teaspoon pure vanilla extract (about 2.5ml)
- - A pinch of salt

Directions:

1. . Rinse the rice under cold water until the water runs clear. This removes excess starch and helps to prevent the rice from becoming too sticky.

2. In a saucepan, combine the rinsed rice, almond milk, sugar, and salt. Bring the mixture to a boil over medium-high heat.
3. Once boiling, reduce the heat to low and let it simmer. Stir the mixture occasionally to ensure it doesn't stick to the bottom of the pan.
4. Continue to cook for about 30-40 minutes, until the rice is tender and the mixture has thickened to a creamy consistency.
5. Remove from heat and stir in the vanilla extract.
6. Allow the pudding to cool for a few minutes. It will continue to thicken as it cools. You can serve it warm, or cover and refrigerate to serve it chilled.

Nutrition: Calories: 230; Fat: 5g; Carbs: 45g; Protein: 5g

Notes and Variations: The rice pudding can be topped with a sprinkle of cinnamon or nutmeg before serving, if desired. It can also be garnished with a handful of low FODMAP fruits like strawberries or blueberries for added flavor and nutrition.

Chocolate Dipped Strawberries

Preparation time: 20 minutes

Chill time: 30 minutes

Servings: 2

Ingredients:

- 12 strawberries (about 200g)
- - 4 ounces dark chocolate, 70% cacao or higher (about 113g)

Directions:

1. Rinse the strawberries and dry them well. Make sure they are completely dry before dipping into the chocolate.
2. Break the dark chocolate into pieces and place them in a microwave-safe bowl.
3. Microwave the chocolate at 20-second intervals, stirring after each interval, until it is fully melted and smooth.
4. Hold each strawberry by the stem or leaves, dip it into the melted chocolate, twirling it around to ensure it is evenly coated. Shake off any excess chocolate.
5. Place the dipped strawberries onto a tray lined with parchment paper.
6. Once all strawberries are dipped, put the tray in the refrigerator for about 30 minutes or until the chocolate is set.

Nutrition: Calories: 270; Fat: 17g; Carbs: 29g; Protein: 4g

Notes and Variations: Make sure to use dark chocolate with a high cocoa percentage (70% or above) as it typically has lower sugar content and is low FODMAP. For added texture and flavor, you can sprinkle the dipped strawberries with shredded coconut or chopped nuts while the chocolate is still wet.

Gluten-Free Blueberry Muffins

Preparation time: 15 minutes

Cooking time: 20-25 minutes

Servings: 12 muffins

Ingredients:

- 1/2 cups gluten-free flour (180g)
- 1/2 cup granulated sugar (100g)
- 1/2 teaspoon salt (3g)
- 2 teaspoons baking powder (10g)
- 1/3 cup vegetable oil (80ml)
- 1 large egg
- 1/3-1/2 cup lactose-free milk (80-120ml, adjust as needed for batter consistency)
- 1 teaspoon pure vanilla extract (5ml)
- 1 cup fresh blueberries (150g)

Directions:

1. Preheat your oven to 400°F (200°C). Line a muffin tin with paper liners or lightly grease it.
2. In a large bowl, mix together the gluten-free flour, sugar, salt, and baking powder.
3. In a separate bowl, whisk together the vegetable oil, egg, lactose-free milk, and vanilla extract.
4. Gradually add the wet ingredients to the dry ingredients and stir until just combined.
5. Gently fold in the fresh blueberries.
6. Divide the batter evenly among the muffin tin cups.
7. Bake for 20-25 minutes or until a toothpick inserted into the center of a muffin comes out clean.
8. Allow the muffins to cool in the tin for 5 minutes, then transfer them to a wire rack to cool completely.

Nutrition: Calories: 150; Fat: 6g; Carbs: 22g; Protein: 2g

Notes and Variations: You can use frozen blueberries if fresh ones aren't available. Just make sure not to thaw them before adding to the batter to prevent them from bleeding color. For a hint of citrus, add the zest of 1 lemon to the batter.

Almond Cookies

Preparation time: 15 minutes

Cooking time: 10-12 minutes

Servings: 12 cookies

Ingredients:

- 2 cups almond flour (200g)
- 1/4 cup maple syrup (60ml)
- 1 large egg
- 1/2 teaspoon baking soda (3g)
- 1 teaspoon vanilla extract (5ml)
- -Pinch of salt

Directions:

1. Preheat your oven to 350°F (175°C). Line a baking sheet with parchment paper.
2. In a mixing bowl, combine almond flour, baking soda, and a pinch of salt.
3. In another bowl, whisk together the egg, maple syrup, and vanilla extract.
4. Gradually add the wet ingredients into the dry ingredients, stirring until a dough forms.
5. Scoop tablespoon-sized portions of dough, roll into balls, and place them on the prepared baking sheet. Flatten each cookie slightly with the back of a spoon or the bottom of a glass.
6. Bake for 10-12 minutes, or until the edges are slightly golden.
7. Allow the cookies to cool on the baking sheet for about 5 minutes, then transfer to a wire rack to cool completely.

Nutrition: Calories: 120; Fat: 9g; Carbs: 7g; Protein: 4g

Notes and Variations: These cookies have a soft and chewy texture. If you prefer them a bit crunchier, leave them in the oven for an extra minute or two, but keep a close eye on them to prevent burning. Add some mix-ins to your dough like chocolate chips or chopped nuts for some added texture and flavor. Just be sure to check that your mix-ins are low FODMAP.

Baked Apples with Oat Filling

Preparation time: 15 minutes + marinating time	Cooking time: 30 minutes	Servings: 2

Ingredients:

- - 2 medium-sized apples
- 1/2 cup gluten-free oats (50g)
- 1 teaspoon cinnamon (3g)
- 2 tablespoons brown sugar (25g)
- 1 tablespoon coconut oil, melted (15ml)

Directions:

1. Preheat your oven to 350°F (175°C). Prepare a small baking dish by lightly greasing it with a bit of coconut oil.
2. Core the apples, making sure not to cut all the way through to the bottom. You want to create a well for the filling.
3. In a bowl, combine the oats, cinnamon, brown sugar, and melted coconut oil.
4. Spoon the oat mixture into the cored apples, pressing down lightly to compact the filling.
5. Place the filled apples in the prepared baking dish.
6. Bake for 30-35 minutes or until the apples are tender and the filling is golden.
7. Let the apples cool for a few minutes before serving.

Nutrition: Calories: 200; Fat: 5g; Carbs: 37g; Protein: 3g

Notes and Variations: Choose firm apples for this recipe as they hold their shape well during baking. Granny Smith or Braeburn are good options. You can replace coconut oil with butter if you tolerate lactose well. For some added flavor, you could also add some raisins or chopped nuts to the oat mixture, as long as you're sure they're low in FODMAPs.

Peanut Butter Banana Ice Cream

Preparation time: 10 minutes	Cooking time: 0 minutes	Servings: 2

Ingredients:

- 2 medium-sized bananas (240g), sliced and frozen
- - 2 tablespoons peanut butter (32g)

Directions:

1. Slice bananas and place in a freezer-safe container. Freeze until solid, usually a few hours or overnight.
2. Once bananas are frozen, place them in a food processor or high-powered blender.
3. Add the peanut butter to the blender.
4. Blend until smooth. This may take a few minutes and you may need to stop to scrape down the sides of the blender occasionally.
5. Serve immediately for a soft-serve ice cream consistency. If you prefer a firmer texture, transfer the ice cream to a lidded container and freeze for at least 2 hours before serving.

Nutrition: Calories: 210; Fat: 8g; Carbs: 32g; Protein: 5g

Notes and Variations: Make sure to use a ripe banana for the sweetest taste. For a chocolate version, add a tablespoon of unsweetened cocoa powder.

Gluten-Free Brownies with Walnuts

Preparation time: 15 minutes	Cooking time: 20-25 minutes	Servings: 9 squares

Ingredients:

- 1/2 cup (115g) unsalted butter
- 1 cup (200g) sugar
- 2 large eggs
- 1 teaspoon (5 ml) pure vanilla extract
- 1/3 cup (40g) unsweetened cocoa powder
- 1/2 cup (70g) gluten-free all-purpose flour
- 1/4 teaspoon (1.5g) salt
- 1/4 teaspoon (1g) baking powder
- 1/2 cup (58g) chopped walnuts

Directions:

1. Preheat your oven to 350°F (175°C) and grease a 9x9-inch baking pan or line it with parchment paper.
2. Melt the butter in a medium-sized saucepan over low heat. Remove the saucepan from the heat, then stir in the sugar, eggs, and vanilla extract.
3. Add the cocoa powder, gluten-free flour, salt, and baking powder to the saucepan. Stir the mixture until it's well combined.
4. Fold in the chopped walnuts, then spread the brownie batter evenly into the prepared baking pan.
5. Bake the brownies in the preheated oven for 20 to 25 minutes, or until a toothpick inserted into the center comes out with a few moist crumbs.
6. Let the brownies cool in the pan before cutting them into squares.

Nutrition: Calories: 220; Fat: 11g; Carbs: 30g; Protein: 3g

Notes and Variations: You can replace the walnuts with other nuts like pecans or almonds or leave them out entirely for a nut-free version. For a dairy-free version, replace the butter with a plant-based butter alternative. For an extra chocolatey treat, you can add 1/2 cup of chocolate chips to the batter.

Poached Pears
with Cinnamon and Star Anise

Preparation time: 15 minutes

Cooking time: 40 minutes

Servings: 2

Ingredients:

- 2 large firm pears
- 4 cups (1 liter) water
- 1 cup (200g) sugar
- 1 cinnamon stick
- 2 star anise
- Peel of 1 lemon

Directions:

1. Peel the pears, leaving the stem intact. Cut a small slice off the bottom of each pear so they will stand upright.
2. In a large saucepan, combine the water, sugar, cinnamon stick, star anise, and lemon peel. Bring to a boil over medium heat, stirring occasionally until sugar is dissolved.
3. Add the pears to the saucepan. Reduce heat to a simmer and cook for about 30 minutes, until the pears are tender when pierced with a knife.
4. Remove the pears from the heat and let them cool in the poaching liquid.
5. Once cooled, you can serve the pears with a drizzle of the poaching liquid.

Nutrition: Calories: 210; Fat: 0g; Carbs: 55g; Protein: 1g

Notes and Variations: If you prefer a more dessert-like dish, serve the poached pears with a dollop of lactose-free yogurt or a scoop of lactose-free vanilla ice cream.

Kiwi and Pineapple Fruit Salad with a Mint Dressing

Preparation time: 15 minutes

Cooking time: 0 minutes

Servings: 2

Ingredients:

- 2 kiwis, peeled and sliced
- 1 cup of pineapple chunks (165g)
- 2 tablespoons of fresh mint leaves, finely chopped
- Juice of 1 lime
- 1 teaspoon of maple syrup (optional)

Directions:

1. In a medium bowl, combine the sliced kiwis and pineapple chunks.
2. In a small bowl, whisk together the finely chopped mint leaves, lime juice, and maple syrup (if using).
3. Drizzle the mint dressing over the fruit and gently toss until the fruit is evenly coated.
4. Serve the fruit salad immediately, or refrigerate for up to 2 hours before serving.

Nutrition: Calories: 120; Fat: 0,5g; Carbs: 30g; Protein: 1g

Notes and Variations: For an additional tropical flavor, you can add some sliced bananas or mango chunks to the salad. If you prefer a sweeter salad, add a touch more maple syrup.

Chocolate Mousse with Raspberries

Preparation time: 20 minutes

Chilling time: 2 hours

Servings: 2

Ingredients:

- 3.5 oz of dark chocolate (100g), finely chopped
- 3 large eggs, separated
- 1 tablespoon of granulated sugar (12.5g)
- 1/2 cup of fresh raspberries (62g) for garnish

Directions:

1. Melt the chocolate in a heatproof bowl set over a pan of gently simmering water, making sure the bowl doesn't touch the water. Once melted, remove from heat and let it cool slightly.

2. In a large bowl, whisk the egg yolks and sugar until pale and creamy.
3. In another clean, dry bowl, whisk the egg whites until they form soft peaks.
4. Gradually fold the cooled melted chocolate into the egg yolk and sugar mixture.
5. Then, gently fold in the egg whites, a third at a time, until fully incorporated.
6. Divide the mousse between two serving glasses and chill in the fridge for at least 2 hours, or until set.
7. When ready to serve, garnish with fresh raspberries on top.

Nutrition: Calories: 350; Fat: 24g; Carbs: 25g; Protein: 8g

Notes and Variations: For a dairy-free version, ensure you choose a dairy-free dark chocolate. To make it more indulgent, serve with a dollop of lactose-free whipped cream.

Almond and Honey Energy Balls

Preparation time: 10 minutes   Chilling time: 30 minutes   Servings: 15 balls

Ingredients:

- 1 cup almond butter (240ml)
- 1/4 cup honey (60ml)
- 1/2 cup gluten-free rolled oats (45g)
- 1/2 cup chopped almonds (60g)
- 2 tablespoons chia seeds (30g)

Directions:

1. In a large bowl, combine almond butter, honey, gluten-free oats, chopped almonds, and chia seeds.
2. Stir until all the ingredients are thoroughly combined. The mixture should be a bit sticky but hold its shape when rolled.
3. Roll the mixture into small balls, about the size of a tablespoon each.
4. Place the energy balls on a baking sheet lined with parchment paper or a silicone mat.
5. Chill the energy balls in the refrigerator for at least 30 minutes, or until firm.
6. Once firm, the energy balls can be transferred to an airtight container and stored in the refrigerator for up to one week.

Nutrition: Calories: 115; Fat: 9g; Carbs: 8g; Protein: 4g

Notes and Variations: You can add other mix-ins to this recipe like dried fruit (in small amounts to keep it low FODMAP), shredded coconut, or other seeds.

Lactose Free Cheesecake with Blueberry Topping Roasted

Preparation time: 30 minutes   Cooking time: 1 hour and 10 minutes   Servings: 8

Ingredients:

For the Crust:

- 1.5 cups gluten-free graham cracker crumbs (150g)
- 6 tablespoons unsalted butter, melted (85g)
- tablespoons sugar (or a low FODMAP sweetener) (30g)

For the Filling:

- 2 cups lactose-free cream cheese (450g)

- 3/4 cup sugar (or a low FODMAP sweetener) (150g)
- 1 teaspoon vanilla extract (5g)
- 3 large eggs

For the Topping:

- 2 cups blueberries, fresh or frozen (300g)
- 2 tablespoons sugar (or a low FODMAP sweetener) (30g)

Directions:

1. Preheat your oven to 325°F (165°C).
2. Mix together the graham cracker crumbs, melted butter, and sugar until well combined. Press the mixture into the bottom of a 9-inch springform pan to form the crust.
3. In a large bowl, beat the cream cheese until smooth. Gradually add the sugar and vanilla, beating until creamy. Add the eggs, one at a time, beating well after each addition.
4. Pour the cream cheese mixture over the crust in the pan. Bake for about 60 minutes, or until the center is set and the top is slightly browned.
5. Allow the cheesecake to cool in the oven with the door open for about 10 minutes, then remove and cool completely on a wire rack.
6. While the cheesecake is cooling, combine the blueberries and sugar in a saucepan over medium heat. Simmer until the blueberries burst and the mixture thickens, about 10 minutes. Allow the compote to cool.
7. Once both the cheesecake and compote are cool, spread the blueberry compote over the cheesecake.
8. Refrigerate for at least 4 hours before serving.

Nutrition: Calories: 450; Fat: 28g; Carbs: 44g; Protein: 8g

Notes and Variations: Substitute blueberries with raspberries or strawberries for a different flavor. For a dairy-free version, use dairy-free cream cheese and butter.

Raspberry Sorbet

Preparation time: 10 minutes

Freezing time: 2-3 hours minutes

Servings: 4

Ingredients:

- 4 cups fresh or frozen raspberries (480g)
- Juice of 1 lemon
- 3/4 cup sugar substitute or a low FODMAP sweetener (150g)

Directions:

1. Place raspberries in a blender or food processor and puree until smooth.
2. Push the puree through a fine-mesh strainer to remove the seeds, collecting the juice in a large bowl.
3. Add the lemon juice and sugar substitute to the bowl and stir until the sugar substitute has completely dissolved.
4. Pour the mixture into a shallow dish and freeze for about 30 minutes.
5. Take the sorbet out of the freezer and stir it with a fork, breaking up any frozen sections. Return to the freezer.
6. Continue to check the sorbet every 30 minutes, stirring each time, until the sorbet is frozen. This process should take about 2-3 hours.
7. When ready to serve, remove the sorbet from the freezer and allow it to sit at room temperature for a few minutes before scooping.

Nutrition: Calories: 90; Fat: 0g; Carbs: 24g; Protein: 1g

Notes and Variations: This sorbet is very tart due to the raspberries and lemon juice. If you prefer a sweeter sorbet, add more sugar substitute. You can serve this sorbet with a mint leaf for added color and a refreshing taste.

Blueberry Compote with Greek Yogurt

Preparation time: 5 minutes	Cooking time: 10 minutes	Servings: 2

Ingredients:

- 2 cups fresh or frozen blueberries (300g)
- 2 tablespoons sugar or a low FODMAP sweetener (24g)
- Juice of half a lemon
- 1 cup lactose-free Greek yogurt (245g)

Directions:

1. Place the blueberries in a saucepan over medium heat. Add the sugar and lemon juice, and stir to combine.
2. Cook the mixture for about 10 minutes, or until the blueberries have burst and the sauce has thickened. Remove from heat and let it cool.
3. Divide the Greek yogurt between two bowls. Top each bowl with half of the blueberry compote.
4. Serve immediately, or refrigerate until ready to serve.

Nutrition: Calories: 220; Fat: 2.5g; Carbs: 42g; Protein: 11g

Notes and Variations: You can also try this recipe with other berries such as strawberries or raspberries.

Strawberry-Banana Sorbet

Preparation time: 10 minutes

Freezing time: 2-3 hours

Servings: 1-2

Ingredients:

- 1 cup strawberries (150g)
- 1 medium ripe banana (118g)
- 1 tablespoon lemon juice (15 ml)

Directions:

1. Place the strawberries, ripe banana, and lemon juice in a blender.
2. Blend until the mixture is smooth.
3. Pour the mixture into a shallow dish and put it in the freezer.
4. Freeze the mixture until it is solid, which should take around 2-3 hours.
5. Once frozen, scoop out the sorbet into bowls and serve immediately.

Nutrition: Calories: 140; Fat: 0.5g; Carbs: 36g; Protein: 2g

Notes and Variations: For a smoother consistency, you can take out the mixture every 30 minutes from the freezer and stir it around before placing it back in the freezer. If you like a sweeter taste, add a tablespoon of maple syrup or a low FODMAP sweetener of your choice.

Raspberry-Smoothie Bowl

Preparation time: 10 minutes

Cooking time: 0 minutes

Servings: 1-2

Ingredients:

- 1 cup raspberries (125g)
- 1 medium ripe banana (118g)
- 1/2 cup unsweetened almond milk (120 ml)
- 1 tablespoon chia seeds (15g)
- A handful of almond slivers (approximately 10g)

Directions:

1. In a blender, add the raspberries, ripe banana, and almond milk. Blend until smooth.
2. Pour the smoothie mixture into a bowl.
3. Top the smoothie with a sprinkle of chia seeds and almond slivers.
4. Enjoy the smoothie bowl immediately for the best taste and texture.

Nutrition: Calories: 235; Fat: 7g; Carbs: 42g; Protein: 6g

Notes and Variations: You can add other low FODMAP fruits or seeds on top for additional texture and flavor. Just make sure to keep portion sizes in mind to maintain the low FODMAP status of the dish. For an extra protein boost, you could add a scoop of low FODMAP, gluten-free protein powder to the blender.

Vanilla Rice Pudding

Preparation time: 5 minutes

Cooking time: 30 minutes

Servings: 2

Ingredients:

- 1/2 cup arborio rice (100g)
- 2 cups low FODMAP milk substitute (like almond milk or lactose-free milk) (500 ml)
- 1/4 cup sugar substitute, or to taste (50g)
- 1 teaspoon pure vanilla extract (5 ml)

Directions:

1. Rinse the arborio rice under cold water until the water runs clear.
2. In a medium saucepan, combine the rinsed rice and the milk substitute. Bring the mixture to a boil over medium-high heat.
3. Once boiling, reduce the heat to low and simmer. Stir occasionally, until the rice is tender and the mixture is creamy. This should take about 20 to 25 minutes.
4. Stir in the sugar substitute and vanilla extract. Cook for another 5 minutes, until the sugar substitute is dissolved.
5. Remove from heat and let the rice pudding cool for a few minutes. It will continue to thicken as it cools.

Nutrition: Calories: 210; Fat: 3g; Carbs: 45g; Protein: 2g

Notes and Variations: Feel free to top your rice pudding with some low FODMAP fruits like strawberries or blueberries. This dish can be served hot or cold, if serving cold, allow the pudding to chill in the refrigerator for at least 2 hours before serving.

Almond Flour Brownies

Preparation time: 15 minutes

Cooking time: 20 minutes

Servings: 16

Ingredients:

- 1 cup Almond Flour
- 1 cup Granulated Sugar (or a suitable low FODMAP sugar substitute)
- 1/2 cup Unsweetened Cocoa Powder
- 1/2 teaspoon Baking Powder
- 1/4 teaspoon Salt
- 3 Large Eggs
- 1/2 cup Melted Coconut Oil
- 1 teaspoon Pure Vanilla Extract

Directions:

1. Preheat your oven to 350°F (175°C). Line an 8-inch square baking pan with parchment paper, letting the excess hang over the sides for easy removal.
2. In a medium bowl, combine the almond flour, sugar, cocoa powder, baking powder, and salt.
3. In another bowl, whisk together the eggs, melted coconut oil, and vanilla extract until well combined.
4. Gradually add the dry ingredients to the wet ingredients, mixing until just combined.
5. Pour the batter into the prepared baking pan, spreading it out evenly.
6. Bake for 20 minutes, or until a toothpick inserted into the center comes out with a few moist crumbs.
7. Allow the brownies to cool completely in the pan, then use the overhanging parchment paper to lift them out.
8. Cut into squares and serve.

Nutrition: Calories: 150; Fat: 10g; Carbs: 13g; Protein: 3g

Notes and Variations: You can always add extras like nuts or chocolate chips, just make sure they are low FODMAP. Also, remember that while these ingredients are low in FODMAPs, portion sizes still matter.

Chocolate-dipped Mandarin Oranges

Preparation time: 15 minutes   Cooling time: 5minutes   Servings: 2

Ingredients:

- 4 mandarin oranges (approximately 320 grams)
- 2 oz dark chocolate (approximately 60 grams),

ensure that it's lactose and dairy-free
- 1 teaspoon coconut oil (approximately 5 grams)

Directions:

1. Peel the mandarins and separate into segments, then place them on a tray lined with parchment paper.
2. In a microwave-safe bowl, add the dark chocolate and coconut oil.
3. Microwave the chocolate and coconut oil for 30 seconds at a time, stirring in between, until the chocolate is completely melted and smooth.
4. Dip half of each mandarin segment into the melted chocolate, then place back onto the tray.
5. Place the tray in the refrigerator for about 10-15 minutes, or until the chocolate is set.

6. Serve the chocolate-dipped mandarin oranges chilled.

Nutrition: Calories: 235; Fat: 11.9g; Carbs: 32.5g; Protein: 2.8g

Notes and Variations: Ensure that the dark chocolate you're using is lactose and dairy-free, as some dark chocolates may contain milk products. If you'd like, you can add a sprinkle of sea salt on the chocolate before it sets for a salty-sweet flavor. You could also zest a bit of the mandarin peel and sprinkle it onto the chocolate before it sets for added flavor and visual appeal.

Low FODMAP Caramel Flan

Preparation time: 15 minutes

Cooking time: 60 minutes

Servings: 4

Ingredients:

- 1 cup granulated sugar (approximately 200 grams) for the caramel
- 1/4 cup water (approximately 60 ml) for the caramel
- 2 cups lactose-free milk (approximately 470 ml)

- 3 large eggs
- 1/2 cup granulated sugar (approximately 100 grams) for the custard
- 1 teaspoon vanilla extract (approximately 5 ml)

Directions:

1. Preheat your oven to 325 degrees Fahrenheit (165 degrees Celsius).
2. In a saucepan over medium heat, combine 1 cup of sugar and 1/4 cup of water. Stir until the sugar dissolves and the mixture turns a golden caramel color. Pour the caramel into a round cake pan, tilting to coat the bottom evenly. Set aside.
3. In another saucepan, heat the lactose-free milk over medium heat until it begins to steam. Do not let it boil.
4. In a separate bowl, whisk together the eggs, 1/2 cup of sugar, and vanilla extract until smooth. Slowly add the heated milk to the egg mixture while whisking continuously.
5. Pour the custard mixture over the caramel in the cake pan. Place the cake pan in a larger baking dish and fill the baking dish with boiling water until it comes halfway up the sides of the cake pan.
6. Bake in the preheated oven for 60 minutes or until the center of the flan is set.
7. Remove from the oven and let cool. Once cool, refrigerate for at least 2 hours.

Nutrition: Calories: 415; Fat: 11g; Carbs: 71g; Protein: 9g

Notes and Variations: Be very careful when making the caramel as it can burn quickly. For a creamier texture, you can replace half of the milk with lactose-free cream.

Cinnamon Rice Cakes

Preparation time: 5 minutes

Cooking time: 0 minutes

Servings: 1

Ingredients:

- 2 rice cakes
- 2 tablespoons almond butter (approximately 30 grams)
- 1/4 teaspoon cinnamon (approximately 0.65 grams)

Directions:

1. Spread 1 tablespoon of almond butter evenly over each rice cake.
2. Sprinkle each rice cake with half of the cinnamon.
3. Serve immediately.

Nutrition: Calories: 210; Fat: 11g; Carbs: 25g; Protein: 5g

Notes and Variations: Feel free to add a drizzle of maple syrup or a sprinkle of chia seeds for extra flavor and texture. Ensure the almond butter you choose is low FODMAP and does not contain any high FODMAP ingredients like honey or high fructose corn syrup.

Berry Parfait

Preparation time: 10 minutes

Cooking time: 0 minutes

Servings: 1

Ingredients:

- 1 cup lactose-free yogurt (approximately 240 grams)
- 1/4 cup gluten-free granola (approximately 30 grams)
- 1/2 cup mixed berries (such as blueberries, raspberries, and strawberries) (approximately 75 grams)

Directions:

1. In a glass or jar, begin by layering 1/3 of the yogurt at the bottom.
2. Add a layer of 1/3 of the granola and 1/3 of the berries.
3. Repeat the layers two more times, ending with a layer of berries on top.
4. Serve immediately, or refrigerate for up to one day before serving.

Nutrition: Calories: 290; Fat: 7g; Carbs: 45g; Protein: 12g

Notes and Variations: Ensure that the granola you use is gluten-free and low FODMAP. Some granolas may contain high FODMAP ingredients like honey, inulin, or high fructose corn syrup. The types of berries used can be varied according to your preference, but be sure to stick to low FODMAP options.

Almond Flour Pancakes

Preparation time: 10 minutes

Cooking time: 15 minutes

Servings: 1-2

Ingredients:

- 1 cup almond flour (approximately 112 grams)
- 2 large eggs
- 1/4 cup almond milk (approximately 60 mL)
- 1 teaspoon vanilla extract (approximately 5 mL)
- 1/2 teaspoon baking powder (approximately 2.5 grams)
- A pinch of salt
- Non-stick cooking spray
- Maple syrup for serving (optional)

Directions:

1. In a bowl, whisk together the almond flour, baking powder, and salt.
2. In another bowl, beat the eggs, then add the almond milk and vanilla extract. Mix until well combined.
3. Gradually add the dry ingredients to the wet ingredients, stirring until the batter is smooth.
4. Heat a non-stick skillet over medium heat and coat lightly with non-stick spray.
5. Spoon batter onto the skillet to form pancakes of your desired size. Cook until the edges start to look set and bubbles form on the surface, then flip and cook until golden brown and cooked through.
6. Serve hot with a drizzle of maple syrup if desired.

Nutrition: Calories: 350; Fat: 30g; Carbs: 12g; Protein: 15g

Notes and Variations: These pancakes are naturally gluten-free thanks to the almond flour. You can add a small amount of a low FODMAP fruit like blueberries or strawberries to the batter if you wish. Be sure to check that your almond milk is free of high FODMAP additives like inulin or high fructose corn syrup.

Chia Seed Pudding

Preparation time: 10 minutes

Resting time: 2 hours or overnight

Servings: 1-2

Ingredients:

- 1/4 cup chia seeds (approximately 40 grams)
- 1 cup almond milk (approximately 240 mL)
- 1-2 tablespoons maple syrup (15-30 mL), or to taste
- 1/2 teaspoon vanilla extract (approximately 2.5 mL)
- A handful of blueberries for topping (optional)

Directions:

1. In a bowl or mason jar, mix together the chia seeds, almond milk, maple syrup, and vanilla extract.
2. Stir well to combine, making sure there are no clumps of chia seeds.
3. Cover the mixture and place in the refrigerator for at least 2 hours, or overnight if possible, to allow the chia seeds to absorb the liquid and create a pudding-like texture.
4. Before serving, give the pudding a good stir and top with blueberries if desired.

Nutrition: Calories: 200; Fat: 10g; Carbs: 23g; Protein: 6g

Notes and Variations: This chia seed pudding is a versatile base for many additions or variations. You can try adding a bit of cinnamon or nutmeg, or top with different low FODMAP fruits. Make sure your almond milk is free of high FODMAP additives like inulin or high fructose corn syrup.

Carrot Cake

Preparation time: 20 minutes

Cooking time: 30 minutes

Servings: 8

Ingredients:

- 2 cups of gluten-free flour (240g)
- 1 cup grated carrots (approximately 120g)
- 1 cup brown sugar (approximately 200g)
- 1/2 cup vegetable oil (approximately 120mL)
- 3 large eggs
- 1/2 cup crushed pineapple, drained (approximately 120g)
- 1 teaspoon baking soda (approximately 5g)
- 1/2 teaspoon baking powder (approximately 2.5g)
- 1/2 teaspoon ground cinnamon (approximately 1.3g)
- 1/4 teaspoon ground nutmeg (optional) (approximately 0.65g)
- 1/4 teaspoon salt (approximately 1.5g)

For the Frosting:

- 1/2 cup lactose-free cream cheese (approximately 115g)
- 1 cup powdered sugar (approximately 120g)
- - 1 teaspoon vanilla extract (approximately 5mL)

Directions:

1. Preheat your oven to 350°F (175°C) and grease a 9-inch round cake pan.
2. In a large bowl, mix together the flour, baking soda, baking powder, cinnamon, nutmeg, and salt.
3. In another bowl, beat together the eggs, brown sugar, and oil until smooth. Stir in the grated carrots and crushed pineapple.
4. Gradually add the dry ingredients to the wet, mixing until just combined.
5. Pour the batter into the prepared cake pan and smooth the top with a spatula.

6. Bake for 25-30 minutes, or until a toothpick inserted into the center comes out clean.
7. While the cake is cooling, make the frosting by beating together the cream cheese, powdered sugar, and vanilla until smooth.
8. Once the cake is completely cooled, spread the frosting on top.

Nutrition: Calories: 350; Fat: 18g; Carbs: 45g; Protein: 6g

Notes and Variations: You can add a handful of chopped walnuts to the batter for a bit of crunch, just ensure to keep the serving size in mind as walnuts are only low FODMAP in small quantities.

Dark Chocolate Truffles

Preparation time: 15 minutes   Chilling time: 2 hours   Servings: 16 truffles

Ingredients:

- 1 cup dark chocolate chips (approximately 175g)
- 1/3 cup lactose-free heavy cream (approximately 80mL)
- 1/4 cup unsweetened cocoa powder (approximately 30g) for dusting

Directions:

1. Heat the lactose-free heavy cream in a small saucepan over medium heat until it just begins to simmer.
2. Remove the cream from the heat and add the dark chocolate chips to the saucepan. Let it sit for 5 minutes to allow the chocolate to melt.
3. Stir the mixture until smooth.
4. Pour the chocolate mixture into a shallow dish and place in the refrigerator. Chill for at least 2 hours or until firm.
5. Once the chocolate is firm, use a melon baller or a small spoon to scoop out the mixture. Roll it into a ball with your hands.
6. Roll each truffle in the cocoa powder to coat, then place them on a lined baking sheet or in a storage container.
7. Store in the refrigerator until ready to serve.

Nutrition: Calories: 90; Fat: 6g; Carbs: 8g; Protein: 1g

Notes and Variations: Ensure your dark chocolate chips are low FODMAP, some brands may contain high FODMAP ingredients such as high fructose corn syrup.

Pineapple Sorbet

Preparation time: 15 minutes   Freezing time: 4-6 hours   Servings: 4

Ingredients:

- 1 medium pineapple (approximately 2 lbs or 900g)
- 1/4 cup granulated sugar (approximately 50g)
- Juice of 1 lime (approximately 30ml)

Directions:

1. Peel the pineapple, remove the core and cut the fruit into chunks.
2. Place the pineapple chunks, sugar, and lime juice into a blender or food processor.
3. Blend until the mixture is smooth.
4. Pour the mixture into a shallow dish and place in the freezer.
5. After about an hour, when the edges start to freeze, stir the mixture with a fork to break up any large ice chunks.
6. Repeat this process every 30 minutes for the next 2-3 hours, or until the sorbet is frozen.
7. Once the sorbet is fully frozen, let it sit at room temperature for a few minutes before scooping to make it easier to serve.

Nutrition: Calories: 138; Fat: 0g; Carbs: 36g; Protein: 1g

Notes and Variations: For a less sweet sorbet, you can reduce the amount of sugar, or substitute with a low FODMAP sweetener like maple syrup or stevia.

Banana Nut Bread

Preparation time: 15 minutes

Cooking time: 60 minutes

Servings: 8

Ingredients:

- 2 cups of unsweetened whole-grain cereal of your choice
- ¼ cup pre-chopped walnuts
- 2 tbsp canola oil
- 2 tbsp Worcestershire sauce
- 1 tsp chili powder
- 1 tsp ground cumin

Directions:

1. 2 cups gluten-free flour (240 grams)
2. 1 teaspoon baking soda (5 grams)
3. 1/4 teaspoon salt (1.5 grams)
4. 1/2 cup unsalted butter, softened (113 grams or 1 stick)
5. 3/4 cup granulated sugar (150 grams)
6. 2 large eggs
7. 1 cup mashed ripe bananas (about 3 medium bananas or 225 grams)
8. 1/3 cup lactose-free yogurt (80 grams)
9. 1 teaspoon vanilla extract (5 ml)
10. 1/2 cup chopped walnuts (58 grams)

Nutrition: Calories: 325; Fat: 17g; Carbs: 40g; Protein: 6g

Notes and Variations: Make sure your bananas are very ripe for the best flavor. You can substitute the walnuts with other low FODMAP nuts like pecans or almonds. For a dairy-free version, use a dairy-free butter substitute and a dairy-free yogurt substitute.

Lemon Poppy Seed Muffin

Preparation time: 15 minutes

Cooking time: 20 minutes

Servings: 12 muffins

Ingredients:

- 2 cups gluten-free flour (240 grams)
- 2 tablespoons poppy seeds (18 grams)
- 1 tablespoon baking powder (14 grams)
- 1/2 teaspoon baking soda (2.5 grams)
- 1/4 teaspoon salt (1.5 grams)

- 1 cup granulated sugar (200 grams)
- 1 cup lactose-free yogurt (240 grams)
- 2 large eggs
- 1/2 cup canola oil (120 ml)
- 1 tablespoon lemon zest (from about 2 lemons)
- 1/4 cup fresh lemon juice (60 ml)

Directions:

1. Preheat your oven to 375°F (190°C). Line a muffin tin with paper liners.
2. In a large bowl, whisk together the gluten-free flour, poppy seeds, baking powder, baking soda, and salt.
3. In a separate bowl, whisk together the sugar, lactose-free yogurt, eggs, canola oil, lemon zest, and lemon juice until smooth.
4. Gradually mix the wet ingredients into the dry ingredients, stirring just until combined. Divide the batter evenly among the muffin cups.
5. Bake for 18-20 minutes, or until the muffins are lightly golden and a toothpick inserted into the center comes out clean.
6. Allow the muffins to cool in the pan for 5 minutes, then transfer them to a wire rack to cool completely

Nutrition: Calories: 215; Fat: 9g; Carbs: 31g; Protein: 4g

Notes and Variations: Make sure to use a gluten-free flour blend that is meant for baking, as not all gluten-free flours will yield the same results. You can also add some chopped nuts or dried fruits that are low in FODMAPs if you like, but keep in mind that this will change the nutrition facts.

30-DAY MEAL PLAN

DAY	BREAKFAST	LUNCH	DINNER	SNACKS/ DESSERTS
1	Banana Pancakes	Grilled Chicken Salad	Baked Cod with Mashed Potatoes and Roasted Carrots	Strawberry Sorbet
	pg.12	*pg.33*	*pg.55*	*pg.76*
2	Veggie Omelet	Rice Noodles with Shrimp	Grilled Tuna Steak with a Sesame and Ginger Marinade	Almond Milk Rice Pudding
	pg.13	*pg.33*	*pg.64*	*pg.76*
3	Quinoa Porridge	Gluten-Free Turkey Wrap	Spaghetti Bolognese with Gluten-Free Pasta Gluten-Free Turkey Wrap	Chocolate Dipped Strawberries
	pg.14	*pg.34*	*pg.58*	*pg.77*
4	Gluten-Free Toast with Almond Butter	Quinoa Salad"	Beef and Vegetable Skewers	Almond Cookies
	pg.14	*pg.35*	*pg.65*	*pg.78*
5	Rice Cakes with Peanut Butter	Rice Paper Rolls with Shrimp	Low FODMAP Vegetable Frittata	Gluten-Free Blueberry Muffins
	pg.16	*pg.38*	*pg.68*	*pg.78*
6	Scrambled Eggs with Chives	Low FODMAP Minestrone Soup	Turkey Tacos	Baked Apples with Oat Filling
	pg.17	*pg.41*	*pg.65*	*pg.79*
7	Buckwheat Pancakes with Strawberries	Baked Salmon with Lemon and Dill	Gluten Free Spaghetti with Marinara Sauce	Peanut Butter Banana Ice Cream

	pg.20	pg.42	pg.55	pg.80
8	Gluten-Free Toast with Avocado and a Poached Egg	Turkey Wrap with Gluten-Free Tortilla, Lettuce and Tomato	Baked Trout with Lemon, served with Quinoa	Poached Pears with Cinnamon and Star Anise
	pg.23	pg.43	pg.61	pg.81
9	Blueberry and Almond Smoothie	Brown Rice Salad with Roasted Vegetables	Sesame Ginger Shrimp Stir-Fry	Kiwi and Pineapple Fruit Salad with a Mint Dressing
	pg.23	pg.44	pg.68	pg.82
10	Tortilla Wrap with Scrambled Eggs and Cheddar Cheese	Lentil Soup with Carrots and Cumin	Lemon and Thyme Roasted Turkey Breast	Chocolate Mousse with Raspberries
	pg.26	pg.45	pg.57	pg.82
11	Lactose-Free Yogurt Parfait	Gluten-Free Pasta Salad with Cherry Tomatoes and Olives	Lambs Chops with Rosemary and Garlic Infused Oil	Almond and Honey Energy Balls
	pg.29	pg.44	pg.58	pg.83
12	Scrambled Tofu	Veggie Tacos”	Lemon and Thyme Roasted Turkey Breast	Lactose-Free Cheesecake with Blueberry Topping Roasted
	pg.30	pg.47	pg.57	pg.83
13	Banana and Coconut Pancakes	Stir-Fried Shrimp with Bell Peppers	Ratatouille with Eggplant, Zucchini, and Tomatoes	Raspberry Sorbet
	pg.31	pg.49	pg.59	pg.84
14	Baked Frittata with Spinach and Tomatoes	Chicken and Rice Soup	Veggie Pizza on a Gluten Free Crust	Blueberry Compote with Greek Yogurt
	pg.27	pg.51	pg.56	pg.85

15	Buckwheat Porridge with Blueberries and Banana Slices	Grilled Chicken Caesar Salad (without Garlic)	Gluten-Free Pasta with Olive Oil, Chili Flakes, and Parmesan Cheese	Strawberry-Banana Sorbet
	pg.27	*pg.40*	*pg.63*	*pg.86*
16	Overnight Chia Pudding with Kiwi and Pineapple	Rice Paper Rolls	Baked Cod with Green Beans	Vanilla Rice Pudding
	pg.24	*pg.51*	*pg.72*	*pg.87*
17	Buckwheat Crepes with Banana and Maple Syrup	Grilled Chicken with Quinoa and Sautéed Zucchini	Low FODMAP Chicken Tacos	Raspberry-Smoothie Bowl
	pg.29	*pg.53*	*pg.67*	*pg.86*
18	Rice Cakes with Peanut Butter	Veggie Quesadilla	Lemon and Herb Roasted Chicken with Steamed Carrots	Almond Flour Brownies
	pg.16	*pg.49*	*pg.63*	*pg.87*
19	Quinoa Porridge with Blueberries and Cinnamon	Chicken and Rice Soup	Tomato and Basil Frittata	Chocolate-dipped Mandarin Oranges
	pg.18	*pg.50*	*pg.71*	*pg.88*
20	Fruit Salad	Egg Salad	Beef and Vegetable Kebabs	Low FODMAP Caramel Flan
	pg.16	*pg.37*	*pg.70*	*pg.89*
21	Rice Cakes with Peanut Butter	Grilled Shrimp Salad with Lemon Dressing	Roasted Chicken with Thyme, served with Mashed Potatoes	Cinnamon Rice Cakes
	pg.16	*pg.40*	*pg.62*	*pg.90*
22	Quinoa Porridge with Blueberries and Cinnamon	Tuna Salad	Gluten-Free Pasta with Olive Oil, Chili Flakes, and Parmesan Cheese	Berry Parfait
	pg.18	*pg.35*	*pg.63*	*pg.90*

23	Scrambled Eggs with Spinach and Feta	Baked Salmon with Lemon and Dill	Ratatouille with Eggplant, Zucchini, and Tomatoes	Almond Flour Pancakes
	pg.19	*pg.42*	*pg.59*	*pg.91*
24	Smoked Salmon and Dill Omelet	Brown Rice Salad with Roasted Vegetables	Turkey Tacos	Chia Seed Pudding
	pg.21	*pg.44*	*pg.65*	*pg.91*
25	Almond Milk Smoothie with Strawberries and Banana	Baked Tilapia with Lemon and Dill	Ginger and Scallion Chicken Stir-Fry	Carrot Cake
	pg.25	*pg.46*	*pg.72*	*pg.92*
26	Baked Frittata with Spinach and Tomatoes	Chicken and Rice Soup	Maple Glazed Salmon with Quinoa and Steamed Vegetables	Dark Chocolate Truffles
	pg.27	*pg.50*	*pg.66*	*pg.93*
27	Banana and Coconut Pancakes	Greek Salad with Olives and Feta	Grilled Tuna Steak with a Sesame and Ginger Marinade	Pineapple Sorbet
	pg.31	*pg.42*	*pg.64*	*pg.93*
28	Veggie Omelet	Brown Rice Salad with Roasted Vegetables"	Beef Stew with Carrots and Parsnips	Banana Nut Bread
	pg.13	*pg.44*	*pg.60*	*pg.94*
29	Blueberry and Almond Smoothie	Caprese Salad	Poached Cod with Parsley Sauce	Lemon Poppy Seed Muffin
	pg.23	*pg.37*	*pg.73*	*pg.95*
30	Lactose-Free Yogurt with Cinnamon and Banana slices	Turkey Wrap with Gluten-Free Tortilla, Lettuce and Tomato	Grilled Steak with Baked Potatoes	Raspberry Sorbet
30	*pg.25*	*pg.43*	*pg.74*	*pg.84*

Conclusion

Life post-FODMAP is not about letting go of all you've learned. Instead, it's about utilizing that knowledge to guide your dietary choices, maintaining balance, and fostering a continued dialogue with your gut. It's about stepping into a lifestyle that considers your unique needs and nourishes not just your body, but also your enjoyment of food.

Here are some key points to consider:

1. Embrace Variety: Celebrate the fact that you can now enjoy a wider array of foods. You've learned your triggers, you know what to avoid and what to limit. Take this opportunity to reintroduce the diversity of colors, textures, and flavors back into your diet. Remember, a diverse diet is often a nutrient-rich one.

2. Mindful Eating and Portion Control: The FODMAP journey has likely made you a more mindful eater. Hold onto this habit. Remember, FODMAPs are cumulative throughout the day - just because a food is low-FODMAP doesn't mean you can eat limitless quantities. Continue to be aware of your body's responses and adjust your portion sizes accordingly.

3. Prioritize Whole Foods: The low-FODMAP diet likely directed you towards natural, unprocessed foods. These whole foods are not only more likely to be low in FODMAPs, but they are also rich in essential nutrients your body needs for overall health. Prioritizing whole foods over processed ones can contribute to a balanced diet and a happy gut.

4. Keep the Food Diary Habit: Your food diary was likely a trusted companion during your FODMAP journey. Keep it around. Continuing to note down what you eat and how you feel can help you identify any changes, new triggers, or evolving patterns over time. It can also ensure you're maintaining dietary variety and balance.

5. Stay Connected with Your Dietitian: Your journey with your dietitian doesn't have to end with the low-FODMAP diet. Regular check-ins can help you navigate this new dietary landscape, ensuring you're not unnecessarily restricting any foods and that you're getting the nutrients you need.

6. Never Stop Listening to Your Gut: Your FODMAP journey has given you a unique insight into your body's language, especially your gut's. Don't let that conversation end. Continue to listen and learn from your body, adjusting your diet to suit your gut's needs and comfort.

7. Exercise and Hydration: While the focus is often on food, remember that regular physical activity and adequate hydration are also key to maintaining gut health and overall well-being.

8. Stress Management: Stress can influence your gut too. Incorporate stress management techniques such as meditation, deep breathing, yoga, or any other activity that helps you relax.

The low-FODMAP diet isn't a one-size-fits-all magic bullet. It's more like a finely-tailored suit, meant to fit the unique contours of your body. It's not about finding a "perfect" diet, but about discovering what works best for your body - learning to listen to it, understanding its signals, and nurturing it in the best way possible.

As you delve deeper into your personal low-FODMAP journey, you may encounter detours or roadblocks. You may find that some foods you love don't love you back, or that some high-FODMAP foods don't actually bother you at all. Embrace these moments as part of the process. They are not failures, but opportunities for learning and adjusting.

Take solace in knowing that you are not alone on this journey. The low-FODMAP community is a vibrant, supportive network of individuals who are navigating the same dietary waters as you. Reach out, share your experiences, and don't be afraid to ask for advice or guidance.

Your Foodlist

Thank you for choosing "The Ultimate Low-FODMAP Diet Cookbook for Beginners." We hope this bonus resource enhances your experience and brings digestive comfort into your daily life.

Each week, as you prepare to embark on your culinary adventure, simply scan the QR code provided with your smartphone. You'll instantly access a week's worth of grocery essentials tailored to the recipes you've selected for that week. It's like having a personal shopping assistant right in your pocket.

How to Use the QR Code

1. Scan It: Open your smartphone's camera and scan the QR code provided in this chapter.

2. Instant Access: Within seconds, you'll have access to your weekly grocery list.

3. Plan Your Meals: Use the list to plan your meals for the week, and you're ready to shop.

Made in United States
North Haven, CT
04 January 2024

47064547R00057